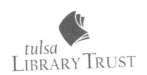

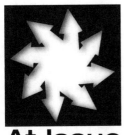

At Issue

Biological and
Chemical Weapons

Other Books in the At Issue Series:

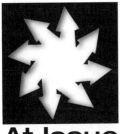

At Issue

Biological and Chemical Weapons

Stefan Kiesbye, Book Editor

GREENHAVEN PRESS
A part of Gale, Cengage Learning

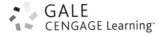

Detroit • New York • San Francisco • New Haven, Conn • Waterville, Maine • London

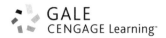

Christine Nasso, *Publisher*
Elizabeth Des Chenes, *Managing Editor*

© 2010 Greenhaven Press, a part of Gale, Cengage Learning.

Gale and Greenhaven Press are registered trademarks used herein under license.

For more information, contact:
Greenhaven Press
27500 Drake Rd.
Farmington Hills, MI 48331-3535
Or you can visit our Internet site at gale.cengage.com

For product information and technology assistance, contact us at

Gale Customer Support, 1-800-877-4253
For permission to use material from this text or product, submit all requests online at www.cengage.com/permissions

Further permissions questions can be e-mailed to permissionrequest@cengage.com

Articles in Greenhaven Press anthologies are often edited for length to meet page requirements. In addition, original titles of these works are changed to clearly present the main thesis and to explicitly indicate the author's opinion. Every effort is made to ensure that Greenhaven Press accurately reflects the original intent of the authors. Every effort has been made to trace the owners of copyrighted material.

Cover Image copyright © Images.com/Corbis.

LIBRARY OF CONGRESS CATALOGING-IN-PUBLICATION DATA

Biological and chemical weapons / Stefan Kiesbye, book editor.
   p. cm. -- (At issue)
Includes bibliographical references and index.
ISBN 978-0-7377-4870-3 (hardcover) -- ISBN 978-0-7377-4871-0 (pbk.)
1. Biological weapons. 2. Chemical weapons. 3. Chemical agents (Munitions).
4. Biological warfare. 5. Chemical warfare. 6. Bioterrorism. I. Kiesbye, Stefan.
UG447.8.B535 2010
358'.3482--dc22
                                                        2010003357

Printed in the United States of America
2 3 4 5 6 7 14 13 12 11 10

Contents

Introduction

Biological and chemical weapons have been used for centuries, even though in today's context we might not think of them as such. In the Stone Age, warriors used poisoned arrows and spears against their enemies. A more recent example occurred in 1763, during the Native American siege of Fort Pitt, when British soldiers conspired to infect the tribes with smallpox by giving them contaminated blankets from the hospital. Whether the blankets were to blame for the outbreak of smallpox among the Native Americans is debated by historians, but the incident is a reminder that warfare by means other than direct combat is an old concept.

The modern use of chemical weapons, however, is barely 100 years old and made its first appearance during World War I, when armies released chlorine gas under favorable weather conditions to fight the enemy. Poisonous gas caused many deaths and introduced a new kind of warfare—one that could take armies by surprise and was difficult to defend against. Soldiers could not defend against what attacked them; once they were able to see or smell the agent, it was generally too late. Protective measures proved mostly useless.

Chemical weapons endure in infamy, largely because they have been an important factor in spreading war from the battlefield to the civilian population. Unlike most bombs or missiles, chemical agents cannot be controlled effectively. During and after World War II, civilian casualties became the norm.

More recently, chemical weapons have gained notoriety by their use not in battle between two countries' armies, but in guerilla-like warfare. The United States used defoliants and riot-control agents during the Vietnam War. American forces sprayed millions of gallons of herbicides, mostly Agent Orange, to defoliate large sections of the countryside and destroy crops. After the end of the war, hundreds of thousands of babies were born with birth defects stemming from these attacks.

The arguably most infamous use of chemical weapons occurred during the Iran-Iraq war of the 1980s, when Saddam Hussein, the Iraqi leader, allegedly used mustard gas and the toxic nerve agent sarin on his own people, when the Kurdish town of Halabja was bombed, killing an estimated 5000–6000 civilians. Iraq claimed that Iranian forces were to blame, but others contended that Saddam Hussein had used the war to exact revenge on oppositional forces within his own borders. In a December 6, 2009 article for the *Associated Press* by Yahja Barzanj, Fatima Mohammed Salih, a survivor, recalls the attack.

The family was at home. There was panic. They first ran into the streets and then went back inside. "We didn't know where to go," she said. "Zimnaku, the 4-month-old, was on my lap and suddenly my older son screamed, saying, 'Mother, I feel like I'm burning.' I tried to help him and my other sons, too. But it was in vain. I saw them dying in front of me. I collapsed, and the next thing I remember is lying in a hospital bed in Tehran."

Another survivor, Dana Nazif, told his story to the *BBC*'s Stuart Hughes in an interview published on March 16, 2003.

"I was 15 years old when the attack happened. There had been shelling for three days so the schools were closed. I fell unconscious when the bombardment started. Most people were in shelters and underground bunkers. When they realised it was a chemical attack they tried to get out, but most of them died in their shelters. . . . In my own family my mother, brother and two of my sisters died. In all, I lost 35 relatives."

The danger of rogue nations using chemical agents is rivaled today by the danger of discarded, lost, or abandoned chemical weapons worldwide, however. They are scattered and buried in forests, on the ocean floor, and in mines. In 2008 phosgene munitions were found in an old range in Hawaii, and in 2007 thirteen unexploded shells filled with liquid were discovered at a World War II training site in Alabama. In the August 2007 issue of *National Defense*, journalist Breanna Wagner writes that accidental discovery of such munitions is a grave concern, "But another more sinister possibility exists. Terrorists could find—and steal—the hazardous containers."

These discarded weapons are known as nonstockpile materiel, meaning nobody knows about their whereabouts, or maintains their safety. Wagner states that "because these weapons are hidden in many unknown places, they are sometimes found purely by accident. Unassuming civilians, such as farmers plowing their fields or children playing in the park, have uncovered them. A group of Washington, D.C. construction workers dug up chemical weapons while building an apartment complex in an upscale neighborhood."

According to Wagner, maybe the greatest challenge for the United States is to locate the approximately 100,000 tons of chemical toxins dropped and discarded along U.S. coasts, in the Baltic and North seas, and near Japan. Dumping nerve agents into the ocean was once deemed safe, but these agents, often stored unsafely in quickly corroding containers, have become time bombs. Furthermore, the Navy doesn't have records of exactly where the nerve agents were dropped. As the result of such dumping, "more than 200 Danish fishermen have inadvertently pulled up mustard gas in fishing nets and been hospitalized."

The threat that nonstockpile weapons could seriously harm civilians—and the even greater threat posed by terrorists acquiring military-grade chemical weapons—makes new efforts to retrieve dumped and abandoned nerve agents an urgent task for decades to come.

Terrorist Organizations Using Chemical Weapons Pose a Severe Threat

Andy Oppenheimer

Andy Oppenheimer is an independent U.K.-based specialist in chemical, biological, radiological, and nuclear weapons; explosives; and counterterrorism. He is the author of the book IRA— The Bombs and the Bullets: A History of Deadly Ingenuity.

While the United States and Russia are dismantling their stockpiles of chemical weapons, the threat of terrorists using chemical weapons to paralyze Western cities and airports is becoming increasingly serious. Transportation hubs are easy targets, and their shutdown due to a terrorist attack could cause great personal and economic damage. The easy access to toxic industrial chemicals and relatively unsophisticated security measures at airports and in subway systems make it hard to defend any country from chemical weapons attacks.

Although the Cold War superpowers are slowly dismantling and disposing of their vast chemical weapons (CWs) arsenals, since 1991 through the outstanding and relentless efforts of the OPCW [Organization for the Prohibition of Chemical Weapons], the military threat from CWs has become increasingly focused on civilian terrorist scenarios and insurgency-prone theatres of war. The most recent examples of insurgent use of CWs were in Iraq in February and March

Andy Oppenheimer, "The Threat of Chemical Weapons: Use by Non-State Actors," *Organisation for the Prohibition of Chemical Weapons*, November 28, 2008. Reproduced by permission.

2007, when canisters of liquefied chlorine were incorporated into vehicle-borne, improvised explosive devices in several attacks, one of which, on 21 February 2007, left several [people] dead and scores suffering from exposure to the dispersed chlorine in an area of Baghdad. In each incident, varying quantities of the chemical agent were used; explosives ruptured the chlorine tanks and dispersed the chemical agent.

Among the heightened threats to transit systems is that of terrorists smuggling toxic substances into airport terminals.

While such a dispersal method is inherently inefficient, [as] much of the potential agent is burned or left oxidised in the ensuing explosion, it nevertheless caused a significant number of casualties, even if the number killed was not enormous, given the quantities of agent present. This illustrates the improvised nature of terrorism and [its] use of weapons primarily to terrorise. Although not efficient in military terms of weapons delivery, such chemical attacks have caused injury, chaos, and psychological damage (especially considering the previous immense suffering caused by CWs to Iraqi civilians). These attacks, however improvised and erratic, show a continued desire on the part of militants to expand their capabilities beyond the use of more conventional weapons.

The Tokyo Sarin Attacks of 1995

Civilian-based CW terrorist attacks are mercifully few. This may be due to lack of expertise and a preference for the tried and tested conventional improvised explosive device (IED). The main precedent is the sarin [a toxic nerve agent] attacks on the Tokyo underground in March 1995 by the Aum Shinrikyo extremist cult. The instant contamination of hundreds of commuters by military-use CWs posed a totally different and more urgent set of response problems on a terrorist prime target—the transit system of a major capital city. That only 12 people were killed was due to the fact that the sarin was not of military grade, but almost 5,000 were exposed and hospitalised, including 135 ambulance workers. During the first 24 hours, 10 people died, nine at the ... site and one just after arrival at hospital. While lessons have been learnt from the incident, most notably improved response and personal protective equipment for first responders, the level of panic and chaos caused by the attacks would likely be repeated if multiple attacks occurred in enclosed spaces such as city subway trains.

Airport Chemical Weapons Threats

Among the heightened threats to transit systems is that of terrorists smuggling toxic substances into airport terminals. While security checks are made before check-in, only at a few airports worldwide are travellers being checked before entering the terminal. A possible scenario can be described as follows: A person enters a typically crowded airport terminal carrying a handbag, walks towards the centre of the terminal, takes a glass bottle out of the bag and throws it on the floor. It breaks, releasing a colourless, odourless liquid. Then the person takes out a small handgun and starts shooting at the passengers standing next to him/her. The guards of the airport respond rapidly and shout at everyone in the terminal to lie on the floor, shoot the person, and ensure he/she is dead. After just a few seconds all the prostrate passengers, including the guards, are experiencing breathing difficulties and nobody understands what is going on. Passengers who are still able to walk start running in different directions. Within minutes there are hundreds of people lying on the floor, injured or dead. Such an event will neutralise the terminal for many days, causing a temporary shutdown of air transportation and substantial economic damage.

Given that security checks are performed before check-in—in the centre of crowded terminals—there is actually no secure way to avoid such an event unless extra security measures are introduced, which could further hold up the travelling public. The response is based on the capabilities of the guards in place and the local first-responder services. Even in advanced countries—for example, the United States of America—the immediate outside response could arrive at the airport after too long a period, i.e. 10 to 30 minutes. In a chemical attack, time is the most important factor for saving lives. Airports must be prepared to respond immediately to any event, until the police assume responsibility. The first response would depend on how much time there is to understand the situation, provide information to the public, wait for the first responders to arrive, ensure they have the capabilities to treat the injured, and prepare the hospitals to deal with large numbers of casualties and decontaminate them.

It is difficult to control chemicals in an unstable country undergoing insurgent attacks, such as Iraq, where there are numerous potential sources of chlorine.

As well as doing their regular jobs, guards equipped with personal protective equipment (PPE) must act as a task force for rescuing injured people from the terminal. An external system would be necessary to check people and luggage before they enter the terminal, a process which could identify, by profiling or advanced technology, the potential or suspected terrorist in advance. These suspects would be checked further in a protected area. Systems are coming on stream [into use] to monitor passengers in waiting areas for chemical warfare agents [and improve] early detection and response. Direct closed circuit television (CCTV) cameras are being installed in areas of sensor activation for instant analysis.

It is difficult to control chemicals in an unstable country undergoing insurgent attacks, such as Iraq, [which has] numerous potential sources of chlorine. And in other developed industrial nations, the chemical industry may not accept measures to restrict the movement and supply of their products. The United Kingdom introduced the Chemical Weapons Act in 1996, and the first prosecution and convictions under the new law, on 24 September 2008, was of directors of a chemical company for failing to notify the Government that their company produced more than one tonne of a chemical controlled under the Convention. In October 2008 a U.S. company in Illinois was fined US $115,000 for exporting a potential chemical weapons precursor, triethanolamine, to Angola, the Bahamas, and the Dominican Republic without obtaining the necessary license. The 11 September 2008 fire in the Channel Tunnel, the cause of which is still to be established and which turned one of Europe's most important transport routes into an enclosed incinerator that destroyed a freight train and all 27 trucks on board, illustrated the dangers of transporting common industrial chemicals.

As in many other countries, basic precautions include keeping bulk access points under proper controls, and monitoring distributions as well as actual chemical warfare agents and certain precursor chemicals banned under the terms of the CWC. The wide availability of toxic industrial chemicals (TICs) poses a universal problem to counterterrorism efforts, which can possibly only be alleviated by individual country legislation and self-regulation by their respective chemical industries, particularly as regards transit both within and across borders.

2

Threats from Chemical and Biological Weapons May Be Overstated

Greg Goebel

Greg Goebel worked as an electronics engineer, but he is writing full time now, publishing his papers on weapons technology and electronics online.

Traditionally, acts of terrorism focused on kidnappings, bombings and hijackings, but within the last decades the threat of terrorist groups using chemical and biological weapons has garnered much attention. As the Tokyo subway attack has shown, highly populated cities are easy targets for attacks and highly vulnerable. The acquisition of military-grade chemical and biological weapons is a difficult task for rogue operators, however, and a successful attack on the general population seems unlikely.

Although terrorism was not unknown in the United States through the 20th century, it wasn't really until the 1980s that the issue began to acquire a higher profile. There had been some domestic terrorism from the left during the late 1960s and into the 1970s, most notably in the form of the "Weather Underground" group, but by the end of that decade the focus had turned towards the right, first in the form of the "Survivalist" movement and then the rightist / white supremacist "militias" that followed them. Religious cult organizations also became a potential domestic terrorist threat. Of

Greg Goebel, "Chemical & Biological Terrorism In The 21st Century," *Vectorsite*, February 2009.

course, leftist domestic terrorism was an active threat in Europe during the 1970s and into the 1980s, in the form of the German "Red Army Faction" and the Italian "Red Brigades," both of which were eventually crushed by the authorities.

International terrorism also came of age in the 1980s. There had been a "dirty little war" between Palestinian terrorists and the Israeli Mossad intelligence organization in the cities of Europe during the 1970s, which was followed in the next decade by the rise of international Islamist terrorism, with the Palestinian issue becoming only a part of the agenda. The story of the rise of modern domestic and international terrorist groups is elaborate and of course not the focus of this document. They are important here because CB [Chemical and Biological] weapons have helped turn them from a serious nuisance to a major threat.

During the 1980s, domestic and international terrorism focused on "traditional" actions, such as kidnappings, assassinations, bombings, and hijackings. Although use of CB weapons by such groups was a possibility, it remained a theoretical issue through the [end of the] decade. The [1991] Gulf War was not only a big wakeup call for the US on the possibility that CB weapons might be used on the battlefield, it also raised the possibility that such weapons might be used on American cities as well.

The Bioweapon Threat

Joshua Lederberg, a Nobel-prize-winning biologist from Stanford University, had been warning for decades that new biological technologies made the prospect of bioweapon attacks much more fearsome. During the Gulf War, Lederberg spoke with government officials, saying that Saddam Hussein's best option for using CB agents was to give them to terrorist groups for attacks on domestic targets. Lederberg was taken seriously, though taking comprehensive action was out of the question given the short notice. An emergency response team was organized at the US Department of Health & Human Services (HHS), and antibiotics were stockpiled in Washington DC.

Lederberg's nightmare scenario didn't happen, but that didn't mean the issue could be forgotten. Rightist domestic terrorists were increasingly active at the time, and Islamists, encouraged by their successful war against the Soviets in Afghanistan during the 1980s, were becoming more ambitious, eager to take on the United States.

On 26 February 1993, Islamic terrorists set off a truck bomb in the underground parking garage of the World Trade Center. The attack was a fizzle, though six people were killed, and the terrorists were arrested with impressive speed and efficiency. The bungled attack bred a degree of public complacency, with the terrorists mocked in op-ed cartoons, but a line had been crossed: Islamic terrorists had conducted their first major operation against a target on American soil. They had failed miserably, but it could be assumed that they would learn from their mistakes and would be back.

The terrorists had actually included a container of hydrogen cyanide with the truck bomb in hopes that the blast would drive the gas up the ventilation system of the building, but the gas was incinerated in the explosion. The threat remained mostly a possibility, and possibilities always end up being lower on the priority queue than active threats.

The Tokyo subway attack was an alert to authorities around the world, and particularly in the United States.

The Tokyo Sarin Attack

The threat became much more active on 20 March 1995, when containers of a liquefied form of sarin [a toxic nerve agent] were placed on five different subway cars on three different lines in the Tokyo subway system and opened by members of a Japanese religious sect named the "Aum Shinrikyo (Supreme Truth.)" Twelve people were killed, and 5,000 required medical attention.

The Aum Shinrikyo sect preached a doctrine that combined elements of Hinduism and Buddhism with apocalyptic prophecies. Japanese authorities quickly arrested its leader, Shoko Asahara, born as Chizuo Matsumoto, and forty other members of the sect. Asahara confessed to the subway attack and other terrorist acts. The Aum Shinrikyo was linked to a 1994 sarin gassing in a residential neighborhood in Matsumoto, Japan, that killed seven people. The attack had been originally shrugged off by the authorities as an accident, caused by a chemical hobbyist who was tinkering with pesticides. That rationalization was implausible, but the idea that somebody wanted to kill large numbers of Japanese citizens at random with nerve gases was even harder to believe. Other acts of terror using chemical weapons that took place in Japan, including the release of phosgene [a colorless, toxic gas] at a train station in Yokohama, remained unresolved.

Investigators found that the Aum Shinrikyo had also attempted to develop bioweapons. Sect members had traveled to Africa in 1992 to obtain samples of the virulent Ebola virus, but [they] returned to Japan empty-handed. In 1993, the cult had attempted to spray anthrax spores off the roof of a building they owned in downtown Tokyo, but they did it in bright daylight, which killed most of the spores, and they didn't have enough for lethal dosages anyway.

The Extremist Threat

The Tokyo subway attack was an alert to authorities around the world, and particularly in the United States. The Aum Shinrikyo sect had planned to carry out other attacks in New York and Washington DC. In fact, the Aum Shinrikyo's attack wasn't the first time extremists had developed or used CB agents in the US. In September 1984, in the US state of Or-

egon, members of a cult community founded by guru Bhagwan Shree Rajneesh responded to a confrontation with the
neighboring town of The Dalles by spreading salmonella bacteria over salad bars and coffee creamers in ten restaurants, as
well as supermarket produce. The idea was to keep voters
home in bed sick during local elections so the guru's people
could vote their own candidates into office. Over 750 people
were affected.

---

*In 1995, Disneyland received a videotape showing two
hands mixing chemicals, along with a note threatening
the theme park.*

The incident didn't attract that much attention, since nasty
salmonella outbreaks happen every now and then in the nor-
mal course of events, and public-health officials concluded
that the outbreak was due to accidental contamination. The
full details didn't come to light until September 1985, when
law-enforcement officials descended on the Rajneesh community, arresting the leaders and interrogating them. They started
singing and outlined the whole mad plot. Several Rajneesh officials received prison sentences of several years, while the
Bhagwan himself was heavily fined, given a suspended sen-
tence, then told to leave the country and not come back.

The salmonella attack hadn't been recognized for what it
was because it was so unprecedented, though citizens of The
Dalles were very suspicious of the cult and believed from the
start that the Rajneeshis had caused the epidemic of food poisoning. Even after the facts came to light, there was a certain
reluctance to discuss the incident in the scientific press for
[fear of] giving other extremist groups ideas.

Obtaining Bioweapons

Rightist extremists were obviously getting the same ideas anyway, with numbers of them arrested for possession of biotox-

ins such as ricin, as well as for working on poison gases and toxins. In 1995, Disneyland received a videotape showing two hands mixing chemicals, along with a note threatening the theme park. No suspect was ever arrested. That same year, a onetime white supremacist named Larry Wayne Harris was convicted of wire fraud when he obtained under false pretenses three vials of the plague bacterium *Yersinia pestis*, which causes bubonic plague. He received probation, though he told reporters he had managed to culture anthrax and said that bioweapons might be a proper response to Federal attacks on anti-government groups: "How many cities are you willing to lose before you back off?"

Following the Tokyo attacks and presented with evidence of home-grown interest in CB weapons, US law enforcement agencies became increasingly worried about a CB attack on a US population center by domestic or foreign extremists. Even the idea that individuals were trying to synthesize CB agents in their garages or basements was enough to cause alarm. The history of the development and manufacture of CB agents is littered with reports of accidents, some of them disastrous. The likelihood of an accident in a basement laboratory would clearly be high, and anyone who would take such a risk was unlikely to be rigorously cautious or prudent.

On 11 September 2001, the issue of a major terrorist attack on a US population center abruptly ceased to be theoretical. Islamic terrorists of the "al-Qaeda" network, led by Saudi terrorist Osama bin Laden, hijacked four airliners on domestic US flights, then flew two of them into the World Trade Center skyscraper towers in New York City and one into the Pentagon. The fourth crashed in the Pennsylvania countryside after a scuffle between the terrorists and the passengers. The Trade Center towers were levelled and a wing of the Pentagon badly damaged. Total casualties from the operation, which was as meticulously planned and executed as it was ruthless, were [more than] 3,000 people.

The attack did not involve CB agents, but in early October 2001, while the dust was still settling from the 11 September attacks, somebody sent off a set of letters to a number of strangers. Within a month five people had died of anthrax, contracted from spores contained in the envelopes that had contained the letters. The five included two postal workers in Washington DC, a New York hospital worker, a Florida photo editor, and an elderly woman in Connecticut. Several others received the envelopes but were saved by prompt medical attention.

Attacks from the Right

The letters used the rhetoric of Islamic militancy, but their intended targets were generally liberals, suggesting a rightist was using the 911 attacks as a cover. The US Federal Bureau of Investigation (FBI) originally zeroed in on Dr. Steven Hatfill, who worked at Fort Detrick, where the strain of anthrax had originated. Hatfill was finally exonerated after being thoroughly raked over the coals; he sued the Justice Department and won a multimillion-dollar award in 2008. Although the Hatfill investigation turned out to be a dead end, the FBI persisted, and in 2007 began to focus on a colleague of Hatfill at Fort Detrick, 62-year-old Dr. Bruce Ivins. The evidence against Ivins began to pile up, and on 29 July 2008, he committed suicide by overdosing on non-prescription drugs.

Ivins' suicide left the Justice Department with the uncomfortable appearance of having hounded a man to death, and in the aftermath a Justice Department spokesman claimed that the evidence against Ivins was conclusive. Ivins had been responsible for the flask, labelled "RMR1029", that contained the specific anthrax strain used in the attacks; all others who might have had access to RMR1029 were cleared; Ivins had the non-trivial technical knowledge required to make use of the spores as a weapon; and during the timeframe of the attacks Ivins spent much more extra time in the labs than he had before or did since. However, nobody could identify any strong motive Ivins might have had to perform the attacks, and statements by some who knew him that he was prone to write threatening letters were contradicted by others familiar with him. [The person who] actually performed the attacks may never be positively identified.

Worries over terrorists poisoning reservoirs or dusting down cities with anthrax or nerve gas are not all that credible.

The anthrax letters were clearly not part of a well-planned terrorist campaign, but the 11 September attacks gave them very high visibility at the time and [gave authorities] an awareness that things could have been much worse. Intelligence obtained from the US military intervention in Afghanistan, the main enclave of al-Qaeda, that followed the terror attacks revealed that the al-Qaeda network was seeking to develop CB agents, and they had already demonstrated that they had the will to use them without restraint. Investigators unraveling the trail of the al-Qaeda terrorists who participated in the 11 September attacks found they had also investigated obtaining use of a crop spraying aircraft, clearly to disperse CB agents over a population center.

Ironically, except for the anthrax letters, the abrupt rise of the Islamic terrorist threat coincided with the near-disappearance of the domestic rightist terrorist threat. After rightist terrorists truck-bombed the Oklahoma City [Alfred P. Murrah] Federal Building in 1995, killing 168 people, the FBI and other US law-enforcement agencies zeroed in on the ultra-violent militias, and militia leadership mostly ended up behind bars. More significantly, although their rank-and-file membership remained generally in circulation, the rightists had predicted that the year 2000 would bring an apocalypse, and when no apocalypse occurred there was widespread disillusionment with the cause. However, although domestic extremists are now keeping a low profile, they haven't disappeared, and the authorities believe the threat could revive at any time. . . .

Dealing with Terrorism

The CB threat can be overstated. Worries over terrorists poisoning reservoirs or dusting down cities with anthrax or nerve gas are not all that credible. A reservoir is very big, and it would take a truckload of toxin to achieve useful concentrations; water quality is monitored, and chlorinated water tends to break down toxins. Crop dusters are designed to distribute pesticides, which are heavy and not supposed to act as aerosols, and so such aircraft would not be effective in distributing finely-powdered bioagents. They could distribute nerve gas, but loading up a crop duster with such fast-acting toxins without killing the pilot before he could get into the air would be very tricky.

Similarly, in 2002 the British Broadcasting Corporation produced a semi-fictional documentary program that depicted terrorists who had deliberately infected themselves with smallpox and then went around in public, leaving a trail of death behind them. Medical authorities familiar with the disease replied that smallpox, while very dangerous, cannot be transmitted by such casual contact; it requires exposure over an extended period of time.

These considerations do not rule out terrorist use of CB weapons, they simply say that such weapons hardly amount to a "poor man's atomic bomb" that could be used to wipe out a city. This is not entirely reassuring, since it is perfectly in the realm of possibility for terrorists to use CB weapons to perform attacks on more limited targets, such as a subway, office building, sports arena, shopping mall, and so on.

Islamic terrorists who were captured and interrogated said that their training in Osama bin Laden's camps in Afghanistan involved exercises in dispersing hydrogen cyanide into the ventilation systems of buildings, which potentially could be a highly effective tactic. There is also the threat that terrorists could target a plant that manufactures dangerous chemicals and sabotage it to spread a huge toxic cloud, much like the 1984 accident at the Union Carbide plant in Bhopal, India, that killed [more than] 2,500 people and permanently injured many more.

Stepping up Countermeasures

US government efforts to confront the threat escalated in step with its rise. In 1995, US President Bill Clinton signed a secret directive organizing existing US agencies for response against a major terrorist attack. This was just a start on a very difficult process, since getting such a large organization as the US Federal government to deal with such difficult problems was clearly not an easy job.

Some things have been accomplished. Unsurprisingly, the government's Centers for Disease Control and Prevention (CDC) is the first line of defense against a CB attack. The CDC has an extensive network of communications with hospitals and doctors, and can both alert them of possible threats and receive intelligence from them about new threats. The CDC has built up a "National Pharmaceutical Stockpile" (NPS) consisting of stores of antibiotics that can be quickly brought from their secret locations to any major population center in the US in a matter of hours. The NPS stockpiles also include atropine injectors, respirators, and other kits for dealing with CW [chemical weapon] attacks.

Serious concerns remain that America is unprepared for a major CB attack. In June 2000, Denver, Colorado, conducted an exercise in which the city was under simulated attack with plague pathogens. City officials were unable to contain the following "epidemic," and the exercise resulted in an estimated 3,700 "cases" and 950 "deaths." It is hard to think of any hospital in the US that could deal with even a thousand anthrax cases, and most would be overwhelmed by a hundred.

Advocates pressed for greater coordination between Federal agencies involved in dealing with terrorist attacks, as well as improved technology to detect CB agents, and funding to medical facilities to give them the means to deal with BW [biological weapon] attacks. The issue remained on the sidelines until 11 September 2001, and then the Bush II Administration established a high-level "Office of Homeland Defense" to coordinate anti-terrorist activities. The complexity of the homeland defense issue has meant that results have been slow to emerge.

For the moment, the subject of CB weapons has gone surprisingly quiet, almost disappearing from the public debate. It seems very unlikely that the issue is going to stay quiet forever.

3

Experts Are Divided over the Risk of a Bio-Terrorist Attack

Marcus Stern

Marcus Stern has worked for Copley News Service in Washington, D.C., since 1983. In 2006, he shared the Pulitzer Prize and George Polk Award for his role in breaking the story of former U.S. Representative Randy "Duke" Cunningham's wide-ranging corruption. Stern has also, in recent years, reported extensively from Iraq and other conflict zones.

Although experts agree that the danger from biological accidents, violence and terrorist attacks has increased in recent years, they disagree on the ways of keeping countries safe from disaster. Experimental scenarios played out after the September 11 attacks overstated the risk of biological weapons available to terrorists, but it remains uncertain how far rogue organizations have progressed and what they are capable of. It is time to educate the public about the real dangers stemming from biological weapons without the scare tactics used before the U.S. invasion of Iraq.

When news of an anthrax attack flashed across American TV screens in September 2001, the public was swept up in a debate that had befuddled government and private researchers for years: What should the United States be doing to protect itself against a bioterrorism attack?

Tara O'Toole, a physician at Johns Hopkins University's Center for Civilian Biodefense [Strategies], thought the attack

Marcus Stern, "Experts Divided Over Risk of Bio-Terrorist Attack," ProPublica.org, December 5, 2008. Reproduced by permission.

was clearly the work of terrorists. Unless the government began promptly investing billions of dollars to defend against bioterrorism, future germ attacks were inevitable and people worldwide could die by the millions. O'Toole, now [Under Secretary for Science and Technology at the Department of Homeland Security], had conducted war games that predicted as much.

Milton Leitenberg, a University of Maryland scholar who has written extensively about nuclear and biological weapons, was skeptical. He thought the likelihood that a terrorist group could have launched such an attack was being overstated. The government should do a thorough analysis of a full range of biological and terrorism threats facing the nation, including balancing the likelihood of a threat with the potential magnitude of its impact, he believed.

Crucial Questions

Now . . . scientists are continuing that debate, leaving the [president] with that same vexing question: What should the United States be doing to protect itself against a bioterrorism attack?

Barack Obama, the first new president since the 2001 anthrax letter attack rattled America so badly, has the opportunity to take a fresh look at some crucial questions:

- Were post-9/11 claims that terrorist groups could develop their own biological weapons of mass destruction overstated?

- Is it more likely that a terrorist group today might get its hands on a deadly biological weapon by exploiting security lapses at the biodefense facilities opening around the nation?

- Even if the likelihood of terrorists obtaining a germ weapon is less than feared, how do you balance those lower odds against the catastrophic and potentially destabilizing impact such an attack might have on the nation?

Just about every expert agrees that the world faces an increasing risk of biological mischief, violence, accident or terror now that advanced genetic research is being conducted in labs around the world, especially China and India. What they disagree about is how to pursue safety without accelerating risk.

"I think in the palace of truth, the scientific community will tell you that the threat of the development of a (terrorist) biological weapon was vastly overblown," said Brian Finlay, a senior associate at the Henry L. Stimson Center, a Washington-based think tank dedicated to reducing the threat of weapons of mass destruction.

But, he added, "the threat of a successful dissemination of a dangerous pathogen has consequences that are potentially so excessively catastrophic that not investing resources to prevent even a remote chance of this occurrence would be an egregious abrogation [negation] of our government's responsibility to protect Americans."

The Legacy of the Cold War

The federal government began worrying in earnest about a biological terror attack in the 1990s, when O'Toole was part of a small group of policy experts that began warning senior government officials of the threat posed by Biopreparat, the Soviet Union's immense secret biological weapons program.

Within 51 days, 3 million people across the United States had been infected, one-third of whom died.

Those experts feared that terrorist groups or rogue nations would recruit poorly paid former Soviet bioweapons scientists, or obtain seed cultures of biological warfare agents from poorly secured laboratories in the former Soviet Union.

The policy experts pressed their case all the way to the Oval Office during President Bill Clinton's second term.

They continued the campaign after George W. Bush took office.

As part of that campaign, a group convened at Andrews Air Force Base in June 2001, three months before the anthrax letter attack, for a two-day war game designed to show what would happen if the United States suffered a smallpox terror attack. Former Sen. Sam Nunn was there. So was former FBI director William Sessions.

In the scripted scenario, dubbed "Dark Winter," a terrorist group released smallpox virus at three locations in Oklahoma. Within 51 days, 3 million people across the United States had been infected, one-third of whom died.

A sequel with a similarly ominous name, "Atlantic Storm," was held in 2005. This time the fictional scenario had an al-Qaeda splinter group use a commercially available dry-powder dispenser to release a preparation of smallpox virus in six U.S. and foreign cities over four days. Again, the outcome was catastrophic.

"The most striking response from the participants in both exercises was that for the most part, they had no idea that something like this was possible," said O'Toole, who helped write the script and direct the exercises.

Overstating the Danger

Leitenberg and other experts said O'Toole's scripted war games greatly exaggerated the ability of terrorist groups to obtain a sample of the smallpox virus (which no longer exists outside defense labs), cultivate it, and convert it into an effective bio-weapon.

"The assumptions that were given for what the terrorists were capable of doing were completely artificial and fantastical," said Leitenberg, who laid out his case in a sharply worded 115-page booklet titled "Assessing the Biological Weapons and

Bioterrorism Threat," which was published by the U.S. Army War College in December 2005. "No known terrorist group in the world has shown the smallest portion of the capability attributed to them in Dark Winter and Atlantic Storm."

But Leitenberg said his more temperate views were largely ignored by journalists and congressional staffers who sought him out for his assessment. They were looking for sensationalist predictions, he believed. "For years and years, it was nothing but screaming: 'It's coming, it's coming.' I wasn't saying, 'It's going to happen tomorrow.' I was saying the opposite."

Seven years after the attack, it seems increasingly likely that Leitenberg's theory was right. There have been no new attacks and the FBI concluded in July [2008] that the sole perpetrator of the 2001 attack was scientist Bruce Ivins, who worked on anthrax vaccines at a U.S. Army biological research center at Fort Detrick, Maryland

---

"In our judgment, America's margin of safety is shrinking, not growing."

Although the evidence pinning the attacks on Ivins is circumstantial, few seriously question the evidence linking the anthrax to his lab. Ivins committed suicide before the government could try to prove its theory in court.

Today [December 2008], O'Toole believes the danger of a mass biological attack by a terrorist group is greater than ever and that huge gaps remain in the country's preparedness. Vastly more money and public attention are needed, she says.

Her views are supported by a congressionally mandated bipartisan task force, which released a report this week [December 2008] predicting that terrorists would use a weapon of mass destruction—most likely a biological weapon—in an attack somewhere in the world by 2013.

"In our judgment, America's margin of safety is shrinking, not growing," the Commission on the Prevention of Weapons of Mass Destruction Proliferation and Terrorism said in its report, *World at Risk*.

Educating the Public

Representative Jane Harman, D-Calif., head of the Homeland Security Subcommittee on Intelligence, Information Sharing and Terrorism Risk Assessment, issued a written response to the report acknowledging the danger of a biological attack but warning, "It's time to retire the fear card."

"We need to educate and inform the American people, not terrify them with alarming details about possible threats to the homeland," Harman said. "While the danger of a terrorist attack using biological, radiological or nuclear weapons is real, preparing the public and training prevention and response teams must be a top priority of the new administration."

Leitenberg believes now, as he did in 2001, that it's highly unlikely that a terrorist group is close to developing a bio-weapon. Every so often, the ... researcher calls scientists and security experts inside and outside government, compiling information that helps him gauge whether ... terrorist groups have made any real progress in developing a bioweapon. In August [2008], when he made a round of checks, the answer was still no. He's still waiting for answers from his latest calls.

The information Leitenberg gathers is by no means definitive—a long history of high-profile intelligence failures bears witness to that. But it is consistent with the views of many scientists who say O'Toole and some political leaders continue to overstate the ease with which a biological weapon can be produced.

"It's a lot easier than putting together an internal-combustion engine," says O'Toole. Critics of the current policy worry that the people who drove the agenda in the [George

W. Bush administration] already have [President] Obama's ear. That would mean little reassessment and even less change, they fear.

"We need a complete top-to-bottom review, a complete reassessment," said Richard H. Ebright, a scientist at the Waksman Institute of Microbiology at Rutgers University in New Jersey. "We need a 180-degree course correction."

4

Threat of Terrorists Using Biological and Chemical Weapons Is Exaggerated

Al Mauroni

Al Mauroni is a senior policy analyst at a defense consulting firm and author of Where Are the WMDs? The Reality of Chem-Bio Threats on the Home Front and the Battlefront.

Before and during the first years of the Iraq invasion in 2003, weapons of mass destruction (WMD) ruled the headlines and received the undivided attention of the government and the public. Biological and chemical weapons, however, have not been addressed specifically since, and the lack of a coherent policy limits a possible response to the threat of nonstate actors using them. And while the threat of an attack on American soil is real, the danger of terrorists seizing military-grade chemicals and staging a large-scale assault is minimal.

In developing the current Quadrennial Defense Review [a study by the U.S. Department of Defense], the [President Barack] Obama administration has decided to move away from the previous strategy of planning to fight and win two nearly simultaneous major combat operations. This is a welcome change, as the Defense Department never had the necessary personnel or resources to effect such a stringent requirement.

Another welcome change is the decision to abandon the [President George W.] Bush administration's quad chart of future threats—traditional, irregular, catastrophic and disruptive—and to focus on conventional, irregular and "hybrid" conflicts.

New Concepts Are Needed

The [George W.] Bush administration placed the mission of combating weapons of mass destruction (WMD) in the catastrophic quarter of its threat chart. This was a convenient way of pushing this strategic issue to the side as it dealt with more urgent and near-term priorities. As a result, the U.S. government did not spend much energy on combating WMD outside of developing agreements to interdict [prohibit] WMD materials and missile systems, establishing the Army's 20th Support Command as the lead for WMD elimination, and bolstering the federal government's ability to respond to terrorist WMD incidents.

> *The arms control community has grappled with the proliferation of NBC [Nuclear, Biological and Chemical] weapons developed by nation-states since 1945.*

Combating WMD was not a priority and was not integrated into traditional or irregular warfare. It was a "special topic." The Obama administration views WMD in much the same way—it remains a special topic for arms control advocates and homeland security officials. There are no new concepts or strategies for how the U.S. government ought to address WMD.

"Counter WMD," the new term, overwhelmingly focuses on nuclear-weapon issues and emphasizes nonproliferation activities. This is unsurprising, considering that the former [Bill] Clinton officials who have joined the Obama administration worked the same issues in the 1990s. It is also disappointing, as it reflects an inability to view nuclear, biological and chemical (NBC) weapons outside of a Cold War paradigm and an inability to realistically address the threat of chemical, biological, radiological and nuclear (CBRN) hazards posed by nonstate actors.

The arms control community has grappled with the proliferation of NBC weapons developed by nation-states since 1945. As the threat of domestic terrorism grew in the 1990s, the U.S. government studied the challenge of responding to terrorist CBRN incidents.

In 1999, the Gilmore Commission's [the informal name for the U.S. Congressional Advisory Panel to Assess Domestic Response Capabilities for Terrorism Involving WMD] first report used the term CBRN because it recognized that WMD was overstating the actual threat. Many analysts and politicians still prefer to continue rhetoric about WMD as "the most dangerous weapons in the hands of the most dangerous people." Yet a closer examination reveals it to be far less ominous.

The Threat of Nonstate Actors

The concept of fourth-generation warfare preceded hybrid warfare—that nonstate actors could significantly challenge nation-states through military operations using decentralized methods and tactics.

Certainly, many examples of this warfare exist—Chechnya, Kosovo, Somalia, post-invasion Iraq, Lebanon and Gaza. Yet military analysts and politicians continue to view NBC weapons and CBRN hazards in terms of third-generation warfare. Any use of chemical, biological or radiological weapons, no matter how small, is considered a mass-destruction situation.

Terrorist groups and insurgents rely on locally available materials and nonstate-affiliated personnel to acquire conventional weapons. At best, terrorist attempts to employ CBRN hazards as weapons will result in small-scale, single attacks with limited casualties.

There is no better example than Iraqi insurgents' failed use of chlorine tanks within vehicle-embedded improvised explosive devices. Those insurgents stopped employing this tactic because it didn't work, yet military analysts point to this singularity and call it the beginning of terrorist WMD ambitions.

It is not easy to obtain military-grade CBRN material, to make military-grade CBRN material or to effectively disperse such agents. Without access to tons of CBR material and a good dispersion system, the capability to cause mass casualties decreases dramatically. If terrorists attempt to develop a WMD-like capability, they will attract much more attention and are liable to be interdicted at multiple points in the process of executing their plot.

Rethinking Terror Threats

Certainly, it is possible to obtain toxic inhalation hazards, develop small amounts of biological toxins, or gain quantities of radiological material and develop improvised methods to disperse them. Nonstate actors can employ improvised CBRN weapons, but these are not WMD capabilities. Nation-state WMD programs are still a significant threat, but we need to stop acting as if nonstate actors can duplicate that threat.

Relying on counter-WMD strategies and military defense equipment that anticipate terrorist use of NBC weapons will not protect the public or armed forces. We need to desegregate counterproliferation, counterterrorism and homeland security responsibilities and strategies. We need to focus on developing discrete [separate] capabilities that address the distinct threats of military NBC weapons and terrorist CBRN hazards.

Most of all, our leadership needs to stop acting afraid of terrorist CBRN incidents—the threat can be addressed easily if we stop using the term "WMD" so frequently and apply risk-management principles and, more importantly, common sense.

5

The Recession Has Weakened the United States' Disaster Preparedness

Thomas Frank

Thomas Frank is a reporter for USA Today, *frequently writing on issues of airport and national security.*

Due to the economic crisis, many states had to cut their budgets for emergency planning and medical supplies needed in case of a biological or chemical attack. Although states' readiness has vastly improved in recent years, the recession could undo much of the progress and put citizens at great risk from flu pandemics and terrorist attacks.

The economic crisis is jeopardizing the nation's ability to handle public-health emergencies and possible bioterrorist attacks, according to government leaders and a new report.

Federal and state governments are cutting programs that help communities respond to disease outbreaks, natural disasters and bioterrorism incidents, and that "could lead to a disaster for the nation's disaster preparedness," a report released Tuesday warns.

"The economic crisis could result in a serious rollback of the progress we've made since Sept. 11, 2001," said Jeffrey Levi, executive director of the Trust for America's Health, a non-partisan research group. Federal funds are down, 11 states have already cut public-health budgets, and more could follow as the economic crisis worsens.

If emergency medical supplies are not maintained or if hospitals can't handle a huge influx of patients, the result will be more deaths and illnesses, Levi said.

The economic crisis in the USA could undo years of investment, planning and research.

Homeland Security Secretary Michael Chertoff underscored the concerns in an interview Tuesday with USA Today editors and reporters. His top concern, Chertoff said, is a "mass event: a big outbreak of plague or some other kind of biological weapon or a nuclear explosion."

"That's the area where the most work needs to be done," said Chertoff, who leaves the post next month. "If we don't consistently invest, we will have a problem."

Chertoff said it's difficult for government and private agencies to spend money to prepare for major attacks "because you're asking people to invest in something that they haven't seen yet—or haven't seen since the anthrax attacks of 2001. Therefore, it seems less urgent than, how do we repair the schools today."

The economic crisis in the USA could undo years of investment, planning and research, the trust said.

In its sixth annual report card rating how well states are prepared to handle health emergencies, the group said "significant progress" has been made since the federal government began giving states and hospitals billions of dollars in 2002.

All 50 states now have a good plan to distribute emergency vaccines, antidotes and medications from federal stockpiles in an emergency, the trust said. In 2005, only seven states had good plans, the trust said.

Richard Besser, the physician who heads the office of terrorism and emergency response at the federal Centers for Disease Control and Prevention, said "incredible accomplishments" have been made equipping states and communities to better handle health disasters. The CDC has given states $6.3 billion in grants. Besser said he shares the trust's concerns "that we could see a decline in the systems that we have built" and echoed the trust's call for more federal funds.

Even with the improvement, preparation varies widely from state to state. The trust says 34 states have bought adequate supplies of antiviral drugs to combat a flu pandemic. But 16 state supplies are inadequate, and some—such as Colorado, Florida and Maine—have minimal doses to give to their residents.

"Where you live will determine whether or not you will survive a flu pandemic," Levi said. He said the federal government should set standards for state emergency health preparation.

The trust also wants states to enact laws that limit the legal liability of businesses, non-profit organizations and health care workers that volunteer to help during a health emergency.

The trust gives the highest rating on preparation to Louisiana, New Hampshire, North Carolina, Virginia and Wisconsin.

The lowest ratings went to Arizona, Connecticut, Florida, Maryland, Montana and Nebraska.

6

Soviet Era Laboratories Might Be Used by Bioterrorists

Sonia Ben Ouagrham-Gormley

Sonia Ben Ouagrham-Gormley is an assistant professor in the Government and Politics Program at George Mason University. She served ten years as a senior research associate at the Monterey Institute of International Studies' Center for Nonproliferation Studies (CNS), and editor-in-chief of the International Export Control Observer, *a monthly newsletter devoted to the analysis of WMD export control issues in the world.*

In the aftermath of the original Cold War, many Soviet-era laboratories known as the anti-plague system have seen heavy budget cuts, layoffs, and lax security. The anti-plague system was once used to fight biological and chemical hazards, as well as to develop toxic nerve agents and other weapons. The fragmentation and collapse of the old system brings about new security challenges for the former Soviet states, as well as the world community. Former employees might sell their expertise to terrorist groups, and laboratories' inventory may fall into the wrong hands. Another challenge is safeguarding the valuable knowledge about biological and chemical weapons and about countermeasures acquired in decades past. It will take a global effort to ensure that toxins and pathogens (biological agents that cause illness or death) remain under state control and that Soviet-era knowledge is used to fight terrorist threats.

The former Soviet anti-plague system stands today as a little-known but profoundly important proliferation challenge facing the international community. The Soviet Union managed this unique system, consisting of more than 80 facilities, to control deadly endemic diseases and to prevent the spread of exotic pathogens. Until recently, however, the anti-plague system's other role—contributing to the Soviet biological weapons program—has been overlooked.

Today, the anti-plague system retains the raw material and knowledge highly sought after by bioterrorists. What's more, more than a decade of fragmentation has resulted in lax security, severely underpaid staff, and virtually no accounting system for highly lethal strains of viruses and bacteria. While international donors have taken some steps to contain the system's physical security threats, existing and prospective nonproliferation efforts are [insufficiently substantial] and somewhat off the mark. Such efforts will not be truly effective until they reinforce the important public health benefits these facilities offer.

Historical Roots

Created by the tsars in the 1890s to respond to numerous outbreaks of plague, the anti-plague system, then composed of 11 laboratories, experienced a dramatic expansion under Soviet rule. By the late 1970s, the system was composed of 87 facilities engaged in disease surveillance, research, production and testing of vaccines and laboratory equipment, and training of civilian and military personnel. The system employed a staff of 14,000, including 7,000 scientists whose expertise broadened beyond plague to other endemic zoonotic [animal diseases that can be transmitted to humans] diseases, such as anthrax, brucellosis, tularemia [diseases with flu-like symptoms and joint-aches], and Congo-Crimean hemorrhagic fever. Most importantly, the anti-plague system stretched beyond Russian borders into Central Asia, the Caucasus, Ukraine, and Moldova, with facilities strategically located in 11 republics.

In the early 1960s, the system, until then primarily engaged in defending the country against endemic and exotic diseases, experienced a profound turning point: it was enlisted to support the Soviet biological weapons program. Initially, anti-plague facilities contributed to the defensive biological weapons program by providing the military with samples of dangerous pathogens, conducting research, training military scientists, and producing vaccines for mobilization purposes. Rapid response teams were also created at anti-plague facilities and were trained to deploy rapidly to an outbreak location in order to determine whether the disease occurred naturally or was the result of a biological attack. In the 1970s, the anti-plague system's involvement in the Soviet biological weapons program went a step further, when selected facilities started contributing to the offensive biological weapons program. This also led to the system's rapid militarization, with military officers appointed to head key anti-plague facilities.

In spite of their biological weapons work, anti-plague facilities preserved their original public health mission of protecting against endemic and imported dangerous diseases.

Three degrees of involvement in the Soviet biological weapons program existed within the anti-plague system. The first, and probably the largest, consisted of a "blind" contribution, [in which] scientists' research was used for the biological weapons program unbeknownst to the researchers. This happened through military monitoring of the work of anti-plague facilities. This process was facilitated by the centralization of research and disease surveillance findings in a central database, and [by] the review of their research findings at two anti-plague institutes in Saratov and Rostov headed by military officers.

The second level of involvement consisted of small teams of researchers working on secret programs in various anti-plague facilities, with only the research team leaders aware of the work's purpose.

A third type of research, concentrated at major anti-plague institutes such as at Saratov, Rostov, and Volgograd, consisted of a more active role in the offensive and defensive programs.

In spite of their biological weapons work, anti-plague facilities preserved their original public health mission of protecting against endemic and imported dangerous diseases. Even at sites that were actively involved in the biological weapons program, civilian and biological weapons work was conducted in parallel but separately. In most cases, biological weapons activities did not adversely affect public health activities.

Post-Soviet Fragmentation

On the eve of the Soviet Union's dissolution [in 1991], the anti-plague system had 89 facilities, including six central institutes, 29 regional anti-plague stations, and 53 field stations located in 11 republics of the [soon-to-be-former] Soviet Union. The system employed about 10,000 personnel, including 2,000 scientists. After the Soviet Union's dissolution, anti-plague facilities were reorganized as independent national networks in each newly independent state, with one facility taking the role of the new network's center.

Yet, the anti-plague system lost its organizational cohesion. Soon after 1992, most ethnic-Russian personnel working at anti-plague facilities in non-Russian former Soviet republics returned to Russia to work at Russian anti-plague facilities or other research institutes. The loss of personnel continued steadily as economic circumstances worsened in the newly independent states.

To make matters worse, conflicts arose in several of these states over the control of the anti-plague system. Some officials favored preserving anti-plague facilities because of their unique experience and knowledge while others sought to integrate anti-plague facilities into the Sanitary Epidemiological System (SES), a network of facilities with more traditional public health responsibilities such as vaccination and sanitation. These conflicts subsided after a 1999 plague outbreak in Kazakhstan made clear the value of the anti-plague facilities. Plans to integrate the anti-plague and SES systems were shelved.

In Soviet times, the sophistication of the anti-plague facilities' security systems depended on their degree of involvement in the biological weapons program.

Nevertheless, this tumultuous period exacerbated the anti-plague facilities' already precarious financial situation. On average, they lost about 50 percent of their budgets and 40 percent of their staff. The scientists that remained received low salaries and irregular payments, which in 2004 ranged from $20 to $100 per month for senior scientists with 25–30 years of experience. With salaries often lower than the regional average, anti-plague facilities have been unable to replace lost personnel with a new generation of specialists.

Proliferation Threats

The resulting proliferation danger is palpable. Foremost is the high risk of brain drain. Considering the undocumented outflow of personnel that began soon after 1992, it is quite possible that some leakage has already occurred. According to anti-plague system directors and veterans, most of the "lost" personnel were technicians and support staff. Fortunately, facilities have generally been able to preserve their scientific personnel, many of whom have passed retirement age. Nonetheless, even personnel still employed by the anti-plague facilities may continue to pose a proliferation threat. These include scientists and technicians with biological weapons knowledge, as well as other scientific personnel who may not have, at least knowingly, worked on the biological weapons program but who possess experience and knowledge of biological weapons' relevance. More particularly, anti-plague scientists are accustomed to working with low-technology equipment and are trained to isolate pathogens in harsh field conditions, often finding their way to natural foci [sites of disease or infection] of dangerous diseases just using their memory. These qualities would be of great interest to criminal or terrorist groups who wish to preserve the secrecy of their activities.

The Soviet Union's dissolution also gravely affected the implementation of security measures at anti-plague facilities. In Soviet times, the sophistication of the anti-plague facilities' security systems depended on their degree of involvement in the biological weapons program. The systems ranged from on-site KGB officers, Ministry of Interior troops guarding facility perimeters, and fences topped with barbed wire to police communication lines and alarm systems with motion detectors on doors and windows, particularly in the pathogen collection rooms.

There were also strict regulations on the storage and transportation of dangerous pathogens. For instance, pathogens were either transported by a special service with armed guards or transferred by at least two members of the scientific staff by car, train, or plane. Strict safety regulations were also imposed for laboratory work with dangerous pathogens. Even though the governments of the newly independent states adopted Soviet-era regulations on safety and security, funding and personnel shortfalls severely affected their implementation. The security systems have collapsed in most facilities. Ministry of Interior and police protection are no longer available; barbed wire on fences are often stolen and sold as scrap metal; alarm systems no longer work due to frequent power cuts and lack of maintenance; and fences have collapsed due to lack of repairs, leaving the territory of these facilities essentially open to intruders.

Security Is Deteriorating

The low level of physical security together with an inadequate accounting system also put at risk anti-plague facilities' collections of pathogens. These constitute a unique historical database of hundreds of strains from various regions of the former Soviet Union assembled over several decades. Although most strains have been isolated from nature, some possess features making them ideal raw materials for biological weapons: high virulence and inherent antibiotic resistance. Yet, pathogens are typically stored in kitchen refrigerators secured with simple locks or wax seals, making them highly vulnerable to diversion or theft. Moreover, vials containing the pathogens are typically labeled, facilitating their identification by intruders. In addition, accounting of pathogens is done on paper logs that are generally stored on bookshelves and could become accessible to intruders.

Another security risk is the absence of background security checks. Without the support of police or security services, most anti-plague facilities abstain from conducting such checks. Many facility directors admit that the only job requirements today for new applicants are "scientific qualifications and good health."

Diversion of pathogens could also occur during pathogen transfers from the natural foci where they are isolated to a field or regional station or during later transfers to central institutes for long-term storage. Neither reliable communications nor any position-location technology exists should emergencies arise. For instance, in the late 1990s an epidemiological team monitoring a plague focus in Kazakhstan's desert got lost and had a serious car accident. Out of radio contact range and without any bearing, several team members succumbed to injuries before their extended absence led to rescue operations. Should incidents occur during transfers, whether they are accidental or malevolent, there is a high probability that the chain of pathogen custody will be broken.

Geography Matters

Roughly 60 anti-plague facilities are located in Central Asia and the Caucasus, which concentrate the largest and most active natural disease foci. This area, however, is the meeting point of all the proliferation chain components: suppliers, established trafficking networks, and potential buyers. It is also a region where borders remain largely unprotected.

Many anti-plague facilities are located on or near the trafficking routes for drugs, small arms, and weapons of mass destruction-related material that cross Central Asia and the Caucasus and proceed northwest through Turkey into Europe.

Several terrorist groups are also active in the region, such as the Islamic Movement of Uzbekistan, which seeks to overthrow the Uzbek president and install an Islamic regime. The wars in neighboring Afghanistan and Iraq have only exacerbated the problem. Moreover, since the Soviet Union's dissolution, political unrest and civil wars have fostered regional instability, as demonstrated by the recent revolutions in Georgia and Kyrgyzstan [in 2003, 2005, and 2010] and public protests in Uzbekistan [in 2005]. This potentially explosive mixture puts anti-plague facilities at greater risk of being caught in factional entanglements and makes them more susceptible to intrusion or theft, with unpredictable proliferation consequences.

To be sure, there have been no indications to date that local terrorist groups have demonstrated an interest in or the capability to use biological weapons. Although there have been numerous outsider facility intrusions over the years, most often they involved intoxicated individuals or people interested in stealing scrap metal. Anecdotal accounts about the theft or attempted insider diversion of pathogens have not led to any known arrests because facility management preferred solving these problems without local police.

Nevertheless, more effective security measures at anti-plague facilities are imperative. In present conditions, dangerous biomaterials, as well as the knowledge and skills of system personnel, are at risk. More particularly, anti-plague specialists' ability to work in a low-technology environment and in field conditions makes them attractive to terrorist groups or states with limited access to high-technology bioequipment. Revelations about Iraq's use of calutrons for electromagnetic separation of uranium isotopes in the 1980s, a technology declassified by the United States in 1949, should serve as a reminder that technologies regarded as obsolete may still pose threats.

International Assistance Wanting

At present [in 2006], the anti-plague system receives little assistance from the international community. Perhaps the most significant contribution, however, has come from the United States through its Cooperative Threat Reduction (CTR) program.

The CTR program currently supports security upgrades at three facilities in Kazakhstan, Uzbekistan, and Georgia. Security upgrades at the anti-plague institute in Almaty, Kazakhstan, transformed a facility with no security features into a secured area with a high [barbed-wire-topped fence], armed guards, motion detectors, and reinforced doors, among other things. Similar upgrades are planned or are under way at the anti-plague institutes in Tashkent, Uzbekistan, and Tbilisi, Georgia. With the recent signature of agreements with Ukraine and Azerbaijan, similar programs will be implemented at two anti-plague facilities in these countries.

To prevent brain drain, CTR has funded five scientific cooperative projects at the same facilities thus far: three at the Almaty institute, which also involves personnel at regional stations, and one each at the Tashkent and Tbilisi institutes. To-gether, these projects employ 52 scientific personnel and deal with dangerous pathogens of public health and security relevance.

Long-standing CTR intentions to implement a Threat Agent Detection and Response (TADR) system also appear to be making some progress. The TADR system aims to create a disease surveillance network composed of central strain repositories and several sentinel laboratories in Kazakhstan, Uzbekistan, and Georgia to furnish early detection of a possible malevolent release of pathogens causing human or animal diseases. State governments, in cooperation with the Department of Defense, will decide which facilities to include in the TADR network. To date, the anti-plague institutes in Almaty, Tashkent, and Tbilisi have been chosen to be central strain repositories in each country, and one anti-plague station in Georgia was selected as a sentinel station. It is not clear yet how many other facilities will be chosen as sentinel laboratories. . . .

Accounting system modernization is also essential; a computerized system would provide fewer opportunities to conceal the movement of pathogens

---

A More Comprehensive and Nuanced Approach

Addressing threats associated with the anti-plague system requires a more comprehensive and nuanced policy composed of measures that simultaneously grapple with security and public health challenges. CTR-funded projects, because they concentrate on a narrow set of security threats, constitute only a small part of this approach. Other agencies in Canada, Europe, the United States, and other Group of Eight members must become engaged to deal with the other security and public health challenges posed by the system. Newly independent state governments must also be involved to ensure that programs funded by the international community will be useful and sustainable in the long term.

Given the current state of the anti-plague system, priority should go to improving security to prohibit unauthorized access to dangerous pathogens. Unlike the traditional one-size-fits-all approach used thus far in the CTR program, tailored security solutions should be implemented depending on a facility's location and size, the character of its pathogen collection, and the activity level of the natural foci it monitors.

All anti-plague facilities have collections of pathogens, but some house temporary collections [and] others retain permanent ones. Central anti-plague facilities in each country serve as national repositories, housing large and permanent collections. These require a complex security system, involving fences, alarm system, guards, video cameras, outside lights, and secured refrigerators to store the pathogens. Accounting system modernization is also essential; a computerized system would provide fewer opportunities to conceal the movement of pathogens. The use of bar codes to replace the existing labels on vials would reinforce the system by making it more difficult for intruders to identify the pathogens.

Regional anti-plague stations, which store pathogens for six months to a year before transferring them to an anti-plague institute, require a lower level of security, primarily composed of secured refrigerators and alarm systems. A computerized accounting system might be useful but not necessary. If the facility is not located in an area that presents specific security concerns, introducing an access-restricting system such as magnetic card access and secure storage for accounting logs will be sufficient.

An even lower security level may be envisioned for stations located at driving distance from the central institutes by providing vehicles and allowing more frequent transfers. Field stations, which store pathogens from a few days to a few weeks, primarily need equipment to secure the pathogens for short periods and during transfers. Local governments may also find innovative solutions to reduce the threat associated with pathogen collections.

In Kazakhstan, for instance, all dangerous pathogens will be consolidated at the central institute. Regional stations will receive simulants [stand-ins] instead to conduct their research work. Such an approach, however, means more frequent transfers of pathogens from regional sites, making secure transfer imperative.

Strategic Considerations

The location of a facility will also affect the type and level of security upgrades. One located in an area where major illicit trafficking occurs regularly, such as in the south of Kazakhstan, or with terrorist activity nearby obviously requires a higher level of security. Similarly, facilities monitoring particularly active natural foci also require a higher degree of security, as they isolate and store a larger number of strains each year.

Reinforcing the chain of pathogen custody during field work and transfers is also an essential task. This can be achieved by providing Global Positioning System receivers, satellite phones, and all-terrain vehicles to enhance secure transportation and foster continuous communications between teams in the field and their facilities.

A second priority is the prevention of brain drain. In this regard, it is important to involve anti-plague specialists in international cooperation projects that will not only support them financially but also use their knowledge to benefit the international community. It is important to engage scientists and technicians who have contributed to the Soviet biological weapons program as well as other anti-plague specialists who, without working on biological weapons programs, still have years of unique knowledge and experience working with dangerous pathogens.

Disease surveillance is also vital. European countries in particular should contribute to such efforts since an epidemic in these states would most likely spread to Europe, as shown by the avian flu and SARS outbreaks recently. In addition, European countries could strengthen the alert and response system by establishing telephone lines to reach local hospitals and doctors in isolated areas. Supporting information campaigns for the local population living on natural foci and training local doctors to recognize the symptoms of endemic dangerous diseases would also improve disease surveillance. These activities were in Soviet times part of the anti-plague system's duties. Today, however, very few facilities have maintained such activities because of the lack of funding.

Using the experience of Soviet-era rapid response teams would also help in the fight against bioterrorism. Their training in identifying the source of an outbreak quickly and deploying an appropriate response would certainly improve the level of preparedness for such events whether in the United States, Europe, or the former Soviet states.

Laboratory Upgrades Are Needed

Besides security upgrades and brain drain prevention, improving laboratory equipment is essential in order to mitigate the consequences of laboratory incidents. Ventilation systems at anti-plague facilities conducting research on dangerous pathogens—regional stations and anti-plague institutes—are desperately needed, especially those located in residential or urban centers. Today, researchers sometimes work with open windows due to the absence of ventilation or air conditioning systems. Upgrades, however, should not lead to excessive reliance on technology. Soviet-era methods, emphasizing rigorous and technique-driven training, should be maintained and encouraged to ensure biosafety.

In these three priority areas, the definition of each anti-plague facility's needs should be the result of discussions among anti-plague representatives; their supervising agency, usually the Ministry of Health; and donor countries. The involvement of health organizations from donor countries in the process is critical to inject a dose of realism in host government expectations, by discussing sustainable options that address both security and public health concerns. Particular national requirements should also be taken into account while identifying present and future needs.

To reinforce security, steps should be taken to establish systems for managing background security checks. Anti-plague specialists should also be educated on proliferation issues and ethics. The Department of State BioIndustry Initiative sponsors such training programs for scientists employed at facilities with BioIndustry Initiative-funded projects; these programs could be extended to anti-plague specialists.

Finally, it is essential to engage Russian anti-plague facilities that still remain closed to international cooperation. Europe and Canada may be better suited to do this because the [U.S.] Defense Department sharply decreased its biological weapons nonproliferation programs in Russia due primarily to failure to sign an implementing agreement with Moscow.

In the end, implementing cooperative threat reduction measures to deal with the former Soviet anti-plague system is necessary but not sufficient to cope with the system's complex dual-use nature. From the outset, the U.S. CTR program has acted in a fireman capacity by trying to put out the most urgent proliferation fires. To be sure, the system merits the CTR program's attention with respect to securing and consolidating dangerous pathogens, preventing their diversion, and forestalling brain drain. Yet, the anti-plague system differs fundamentally from other threat reduction challenges in that it has had and still assumes a critically important public health role. This capacity desperately needs to be sharpened if the international community is [to cope effectively] with the prospects of future and perhaps global epidemics.

7

The Government Needs to Prevent Abuse of Biological Research

Stephen Maurer

Stephen Maurer is an adjunct associate professor at the University of California, Berkeley's Goldman School of Public Policy and director of the Goldman School Project on Information Technology and Homeland Security. His research focuses on the security, innovation, and antitrust implications of synthetic biology and other cutting-edge science. Maurer is also the editor of the book WMD Terrorism: Science and Policy Choices.

Modern technology has enabled scientists to recreate old viruses and develop new ones from scratch. And while the trade of DNA and genes is flourishing, security and regulations hardly exist. More effective than any government program trying to rein in the burgeoning industry, however, are in-house screenings at biocompanies as well as self-regulation. The key to success is to create a database that enables companies worldwide to share information about clients and potential dangers. The government needs to support existing industry programs to reduce the risk of terrorists and rogue nations gaining access to deadly viruses and pathogens.

Governments trying to prevent the misuse of biological research face considerable challenges. The technologies needed to create biological weapons are freely available at aca-

Stephen Maurer, "Grassroots Efforts to Impede Bioterrorism," *Bulletin of the Atomic Scientists*, March 5, 2009. Reproduced by permission of Bulletin of the Atomic Scientists: The Magazine of Global Security News & Analysis.

demic laboratories and biotech companies around the world, and researchers are constantly trading information through a complex web of open science networks and markets. Trying to identify, much less monitor or control these activities, seems hopeless. How, then, should society keep biological information and technologies out of the hands of terrorists?

A New Approach

The old Cold War methods tried to control science and markets from the outside. Given the power of these institutions, though, it probably makes more sense to enlist them as partners. That's the approach my project at the University of California, Berkeley is taking to make one of biology's fastest growing fields—synthetic biology—safer.

Over the past decade, synthetic biologists have used artificial DNA to revive extinct viruses (e.g. 1918 influenza) and create radically new and reengineered organisms. Shortly after 9/11, researchers and industry began asking themselves what could be done to keep this power away from terrorists. Strikingly, many of the best ideas didn't require government intervention at all. Last April [2008], synthetic biology's leading trade association, the Industry Association Synthetic Biology (IASB), held a meeting in Munich to select the best ideas and organize grassroots initiatives to launch them. Now, nearly a year later, these projects are starting to take off.

Existing screening software routinely identifies large numbers of harmless genes which human experts must then examine before an order can be filled.

Keeping Terrorists out of the Market

The simplest but most immediate threat is that terrorists could use synthetic biology to manufacture otherwise unobtainable pathogens such as 1918 influenza or smallpox. Fortunately, most companies that make synthetic DNA already screen incoming orders against the so-called select agent list of pathogens. The problem is that different companies have different screening procedures, and a few companies do no screening at all. Addressing these problems with an international treaty would take decades. Can a market-based solution do better?

The executives who run the new gene synthesis companies readily admit that customers want them to screen and are often indignant when they don't. The fact that most companies already screen is encouraging: However imperfectly, consumers' preferences must be getting through! The task now is to make these market signals even stronger. In practice, this means designing shrewd initiatives so that customers will know immediately when a supplier's screening program is inadequate and, if necessary, take their business elsewhere.

IASB has made this strategy its top priority. The basic idea is to develop a seal of approval that customers can consult. This, in turn, will require an agreed code of conduct that defines responsible screening. IASB's current draft of a code is ambitious and will require most companies to upgrade their programs. Members expect to finalize the document in July [the code was finalized in November 2009].

Improving Screening Software

Existing screening software routinely identifies large numbers of harmless genes which human experts must then examine before an order can be filled. This makes it impractical to screen for threats beyond the relatively short list of select agents. The day is coming, though, when companies will also need to screen for short DNA sequences ("oligos") and/or genetically engineered threats that look radically different from any known organism. Some observers have argued that government should set standards for this next-generation screening software—or even try to write it. But nobody really knows what such a program would look like.

Fortunately, gene synthesis companies have learned a great deal from operating first-generation screening programs. The first step to improving screening software, therefore, will be to break down confidentiality so that companies can pool what they know. Several IASB members have already agreed to get the ball rolling by publishing their experiences. Thereafter, Berkeley and IASB plan to establish a password-protected site where companies can share information with each other and, in many cases, the public.

The biggest technological challenge will be to create a comprehensive database that says whether genes are harmful ("virulent") or benign. This is a large undertaking and will almost certainly need government support in the long run. For now, though, IASB has found a way to get started. Member companies already pay employees to search the scientific literature for evidence of virulence each time their screening software identifies suspicious genes. This information is usually discarded, but preserving and sharing it would save money for everyone. (Corporate open-source software collaborations routinely follow this logic when they share the work of developing web servers and other projects.) The key is to create a state-of-the-art bioinformatics depository where this sharing can take place. IASB's Markus Fischer is working with Berkeley to make this open source biosecurity project a reality. We expect to have a basic version of the site, known as VIREP, on line by early 2010 [at www.virep.org]. Several IASB members have already agreed to donate virulence data.

Experiments of Concern

Improved screening will provide a reasonable hedge against synthetic biology's most immediate threats. In the long run, though, it is worth asking whether today's state-of-the-art biology experiments could inadvertently make advanced weapons more lethal or easier to acquire. Deciding which of these "experiments of concern" should go forward will be difficult. Furthermore, the fact that most projects offer benefits as well as dangers means that the decision won't be easy. The problem associated with experiments of concern, at least for now, is that no one really knows what they look like or can write down any clear principles for deciding which ones should go forward. Common law courts the world over routinely make case-by-case decisions on the theory that principles will eventually emerge later. Synthetic biology will almost certainly have to follow this same strategy.

My Berkeley project is working to develop an online portal where scientists, Institutional Biosafety Committees, and other interested parties can get quick, expert, and impartial advice about whether "experiments of concern" should go forward. The project's information technology manager Jason Christopher has spent much of the last year working with a commercial developer to write software for the portal and is now in the process of testing it. (The software will be freely available.) Early support from the synthetic biology and security communities has been impressive, with two dozen experts already volunteering to serve as reviewers.

More than most people, synthetic biologists know that progress is impossible without trial, error, and a willingness to fail.

The acid test will be seeing how many community members ask for advice. Here too, there is reason to be optimistic. The principle of seeking sanity checks before embarking on experiments of concern is already well-established in synthetic biology, most notably in *Science*'s 2005 decision to obtain informal review from [then-]CDC director Julie Gerberding before running a paper announcing that the 1918 influenza virus had been artificially synthesized. Furthermore, two anonymous scientists have already agreed to submit their experiments to the portal as part of a trial run. Following this trial, the portal's web site will begin taking inquiries from scientists and biosafety committees all over the world. Each new query will be examined by a panel of three volunteers, including at least one biologist and one biosecurity expert. Most inquiries should receive a detailed response within two weeks.

What Government Can Do

It is not too soon to ask how government can coordinate and build on these grassroots efforts. The simplest option would be for government to make some voluntary measures mandatory. For example, U.S. authorities are considering draft regulations that would require federal grantees to follow the existing norm against doing business with gene synthesis companies that fail to screen orders. In some cases, though, it may also make sense for government to defer some regulation until the community has had a chance to find out which new ideas (notably the portal and next-generation screening software) work and which don't. Finally, government should consider imaginative partnerships with existing industry efforts so that projects such as VIREP can go even further.

Synthetic biologists' efforts to improve security at the community level are just beginning. The important thing, though, is that the community has turned the corner from talk to action. More than most people, synthetic biologists know that progress is impossible without trial, error, and a willingness to fail. Government could do much worse than to follow their example.

8

The U.S. Is Struggling to Destroy Its Chemical Weapons

Bob Drogin

Bob Drogin covers national security and intelligence for the Los Angeles Times. *He previously served as a foreign correspondent for the* Times *in Asia and Africa, and as a national correspondent based in New York. He has won or shared multiple journalism awards, among them the Pulitzer Prize, the Robert F. Kennedy Journalism Award, and the George Polk Award. He is the author of* Spies, Lies, and the Man Behind Them: How America Went to War in Iraq.

Despite efforts to destroy America's stockpile of chemical weapons, the United States, after long years of delays and technical problems, is far behind its schedule set by treaties and federal law. Sites disposing of hazardous material have been beset with mistakes and accidents, which might threaten the environment and civilian population. Currently on pace to finish the work by 2021, the United States is in danger of breaching international treaties calling for a 2017 deadline, thus jeopardizing the goodwill and compliance of other nations.

Behind armed guards in bulletproof booths deep in the Kentucky woods, workers have begun pouring the foundations for a $3 billion complex designed to destroy America's last stockpile of deadly chemical weapons.

The aging arsenal at the Blue Grass Army Depot contains 523 tons of liquid VX and sarin—lethal nerve agents produced during the Cold War—and mustard, a blister agent that caused horrific casualties in World War I. The [President Barack] Obama administration has pushed to speed up the disposal operation after decades of delay, skyrocketing costs and daunting technical problems. The arms must be destroyed by April 2012 under international treaty and by December 2017 under federal law. But the Pentagon notified Congress in May that, even under what it called an accelerated schedule, it would not finish the job until 2021.

A senior Obama administration aide downplayed the diplomatic fallout of missing the arms control deadline.

"No one accuses the United States of willfully seeking to violate the treaty for purposes of maintaining our chemical weapons arsenal," said Gary Samore, the White House coordinator for weapons of mass destruction. "Everyone understands this is a technical problem."

For now, more than 100,000 poison-filled munitions are stacked like bottles of wine in 44 dirt-covered concrete bunkers beside the construction site. Intruders are kept out by a double row of chain-link fences topped with cameras, coiled razor wire, and signs warning, "Use of Deadly Force Authorized."

About a third of the World War II-era igloos are so dilapidated that green plastic sheeting was recently draped over them to keep the rain out. Some of the rockets, warheads, mortar rounds and artillery shells inside are just as old—and are leaking as well.

On Monday [August 17, 2009], trace amounts of mustard vapor were detected inside a munitions bunker. That followed a sarin leak in another igloo in June [2009] and separate sarin and mustard leaks in May [2009].

"We do experience leakers from time to time at very, very low levels," said Lieutenant Colonel David Musgrave, commander of the Blue Grass Chemical Activity, as the storage site is called. He said no toxic plumes have escaped the igloos or threatened the surrounding community.

Local emergency response officials, however, have stepped up precautions.

Madison County recently obtained federal funds to give 40,000 special radios to residents and businesses here in the lush, rolling hills of central Kentucky, home to horse farms and tobacco fields. The radios will sound an alarm if a major accident occurs.

"I'm happier now," said Kent Clark, the county judge-executive. "People have finally stood up and noticed that we live next to the country's deadliest stockpile."

Blue Grass is one of six Army installations where chemical weapons are stored. Four are incinerating their stockpiles. In the 1980s, Pentagon officials estimated a $600 million price tag to eliminate the toxic arsenals. The estimated cost today: $40 billion.

"We wound up having to build many more destruction facilities than originally planned," said Milton Leitenberg, a weapons expert at the University of Maryland. "The more time it takes, the more it costs."

Blue Grass is the last site to store lethal VX and sarin and will be the last to destroy its weapons. The task is unusually difficult because, unlike other sites, all the chemicals here are loaded in highly explosive M55 rockets and corroding, fully armed munitions.

"It's like super toxic hazardous waste at this point," said Jonathan Tucker, a nonproliferation specialist at the Monterey Institute of International Studies. "Getting rid of it is a very nasty process."

Concerns about safety at Blue Grass were highlighted last month when lawyers for Donald Van Winkle—a former chemical weapons monitor who claims he was forced out after he uncovered unsafe conditions—obtained an Army investigative report through the Freedom of Information Act.

The Inspector General's report confirmed Van Winkle's charge that a key air monitoring component was improperly installed in the VX igloos between September 2003 and August 2005.

VX is the deadliest of all nerve agents.

An "accurate measurement of any VX agent vapor release would not have been possible," the 51-page report concluded. It found "no evidence" that VX had leaked or endangered the public before the error was corrected.

In December [2008], a federal administrative law judge dismissed Van Winkle's whistle-blower lawsuit against the Army. The 38-year-old Persian Gulf war veteran remains bitter about his attempts to expose what he said were dangerous conditions.

Inspectors noted unsafe storage and disposal of hazardous material, inaccurate record keeping and inadequate training "to prevent releases of chemical warfare agents to the environment."

"I tried to protect a place that's crucial to national security," Van Winkle said. "I thought they'd thank me."

Another self-described whistle-blower, Kim Schafermeyer, 59, claimed he was fired as a chemist in 2006 in retaliation for citing safety and pollution problems at Blue Grass. A judge dismissed his lawsuit last year on a technicality.

Schafermeyer contends the aging munitions are decomposing faster than officials admit. "They are highly unstable," he said. "These things should be destroyed next week."

Documented problems at the facility have persisted.

In October 2007, the Kentucky Department of Environmental Protection cited Blue Grass for four violations of state regulations. Inspectors noted unsafe storage and disposal of hazardous material, inaccurate record keeping and inadequate training "to prevent releases of chemical warfare agents to the environment."

Partly as a result, the environmental crimes section at the U.S. Justice Department launched a criminal investigation. The grand jury probe concluded in April [2009] without any indictments or arrests, Blue Grass legal counsel B. Kevin Bennett said.

By the mid-1980s, the Army had stockpiled 31,500 tons of liquid chemical agents in eight states and on Johnston Atoll, a remote Pacific island.

U.S. forces have not fired chemical munitions in combat since World War I, although the Air Force during the Vietnam War sprayed Agent Orange and other herbicides to defoliate jungles and crop lands. The post-war Vietnamese government said the defoliants caused thousands of deaths, disabilities and birth defects. Some U.S. soldiers also were affected, and the Veterans Affairs Department has listed numerous cancers and other illnesses as "presumptive" conditions of Agent Orange exposure.

In 1975, President Gerald Ford signed the Geneva Protocol, a treaty that prohibits first use of chemical weapons. But the Pentagon continued to produce deadly nerve agents in battlefield weapons as a deterrent—or in case the Cold War turned hot.

By the mid-1980s, the Army had stockpiled 31,500 tons of liquid chemical agents in eight states and on Johnston Atoll, a remote Pacific island.

But political pressure was growing to get rid of the witch's brew. In 1986, President Ronald Reagan signed a law to eliminate chemical warfare material and production facilities. Officials vowed to complete the disarmament by 1994.

The program instead sparked bitter political battles.

The Pentagon and the National Academy of Sciences insisted incineration was the easiest, cheapest and safest solution. But local activists and environmental groups opposed moving the munitions or incinerating them at each site, arguing neither option was safe.

The first incinerator began operating at Johnston Atoll in 1990. It completed the job and closed a decade later as debate continued to rage at other sites.

"We sued everyone we could," said Craig Williams, a Vietnam veteran who heads the Chemical Weapons Working Group, an anti-incineration coalition based above a quilt shop in Berea, Kentucky, near Blue Grass.

The logjam broke after Sept. 11, 2001, when homeland security officials warned that the igloos made tempting targets for terrorists. Alabama, Arkansas, Oregon and Utah soon began incinerating their stockpiles.

On Wednesday [August 19, 2009], a federal judge in Washington tossed out a lawsuit from Williams' group that sought to close the four incinerators for allegedly pumping out hazardous emissions. The judge ruled that the Army had proved the incinerators were safe.

"On the whole, they (have) worked pretty well," said Paul Walker, head of Global Green USA, a nonproliferation group. "From time to time, they would burp out live agent and had toxic releases. But no one was injured."

Under pressure from incineration opponents, however, Congress ordered the Pentagon to seek other options. The result: machines in sealed chambers that disassemble the munitions, neutralize the toxic chemicals inside and decontaminate the waste.

"These facilities are expensive because they're essentially operated by robots," Tucker said.

Disposal operations using those techniques recently concluded in Indiana and Maryland, and the Pentagon says 60 percent of the U.S. arsenal is now destroyed.

The Obama administration has stepped up funding to push the process. Last month [July 2009], the House approved $547 million for the last two disposal facilities at Blue Grass and the Pueblo Chemical Depot in Colorado. If the Senate agrees, it would be a sharp increase from previous years.

Under the defense appropriations bill passed last year [2008], the Pentagon must complete destruction of the U.S. chemical weapons stockpile "in no circumstances later than" Dec. 31, 2017. However, under the timetable sent to Congress in May [2009], Blue Grass won't begin operations until 2018 and won't finish destroying the munitions for three years.

It thus is on track to violate a deadline set by the Chemical Weapons Convention, an international treaty that requires signatories to eliminate their stockpiles by 2007.

Washington has obtained a five-year extension, but the treaty doesn't provide for a second deferral. U.S. diplomats recently visited The Hague, where the treaty organization is based, to explain the problem.

"We're going to take all sorts of whacks from other delegations, especially the Iranians," Walker said. "How can the U.S. expect other countries to honor the treaty if we're in violation?"

For now, crews are busy at an 18-acre site carved into the forest at Blue Grass. On a recent muggy afternoon, they operated front-end loaders and laid pipe. A red steel crane towered overhead. It will help erect a six-story building designed to contain the accidental detonation of poison-filled rockets or other munitions.

"No vapors would get out and there'd be no breaches to the wall," said Mark Seely, the project manager.

Nearby, row after row of chemical weapons igloos were visible in a grassy field, patrolled by armed guards in a white pickup truck.

"This facility is not (like building) a shopping mall," Seely said. "It's one of a kind."

9

Off-Shore Chemical Weapons Dump Sites May Pose a Great Risk

Nicole Branan

Nicole Branan is a contributing writer to EARTH magazine, a monthly magazine devoted to earth science, energy and environment news.

After World War II, many chemical weapons were dumped in the Atlantic and Pacific oceans. Sometimes, the barrels with toxins were not properly sealed, but even leftover bombs and once secure containers have corroded and threaten to poison the waters. Search teams not only face the problem of locating the dumping sites, which are hard to spot due to general dumping and shipwrecks, but they also lack proper means to rescue the chemical. Therefore, any attempt to lift old nerve agents and toxins might cause a disaster.

Flash back to 1944: It's a misty Hawaiian morning and a military vessel carries a nervous crew and deadly cargo from Pearl Harbor into the Pacific. The crew's instructions are clear: Travel eight kilometers out to sea and dump tons of unused chemical weapons that are piled on deck. As the ship reaches the open ocean, the captain slows the vessel and sailors start pushing their lethal freight into the water. During the next half-hour, several thousand chemical bombs go overboard and into the abyss.

Today, such a scenario seems unimaginable. But between the early 20th century and the mid-1970s, many nations used the deep ocean floor as a dumping ground for leftover bombs filled with chemicals such as chemical mustard, lewisite, sarin and tabun. Times—and mind-sets—were different then. The seafloor was considered an inaccessible place that no one would ever lay eyes on. And countries around the world faced a tough problem: Two world wars had left behind untold amounts of dangerous weapons that no one knew how to safely destroy.

Throwing this dangerous garbage into the deep sea seemed like a reasonable and safe solution. Between the end of World War I and 1975, when the Convention on the Prevention of Marine Pollution by Dumping of Wastes and Other Matter came into force, the militaries of many nations dumped several hundred thousand tons of chemical weapons into various parts of the world's oceans, including some 30 sites off U.S. shores, including the Mid-Atlantic and Hawaii. Since then, these weapons, along with the containers that hold them, have quietly rotted away on the seafloor. What that rotting means for the environment remains unknown.

Now a team of researchers at the University of Hawaii at Mānoa is embarking on the most comprehensive study to date to examine a chemical weapons dump site in U.S. waters. The Hawaii Undersea Munitions and Material Assessment study, which is funded by the U.S. Army, will look for chemical weapons south of Pearl Harbor off the coast of Oahu. The work could help establish protocols for similar studies in the future, the researchers say.

The team's target is one of at least three known chemical warfare dumping sites around the Hawaiian Islands. According to historical records, 16,000 chemical mustard bombs were dumped in the area. The study's first objective is to find them, says Roy Wilkens of the Hawaii Institute of Geophysics and Planetology in Honolulu. He and his team surveyed a 60-

square-kilometer patch of the seafloor using sonar technology last year. Their data generated maps that yielded some "target areas," Wilkens says, that the team will explore with cameras, manned research submersibles and remotely operated vehicles in the coming months.

Looking for specific weapons, some of which are in corroded metal containers that are likely overgrown with vegetation, is tough because the seafloor around Pearl Harbor is anything but pristine. "The place is littered with everything from sunken ships to World War II airplanes," Wilkens says. During a routine equipment test in the 1990s, he and his team even came across old American Standard toilets—apparently surplus left over after the war. It's hard to tell a sonar blip generated by a container full of chemical weapons from that of other garbage, says Margo Edwards of the Hawaii Institute of Geophysics and Planetology. "So, whether our target areas are weapons or fields of toilets, we won't know until we go down there with cameras."

Once they locate the weapons, the team plans to test for degradation products—compounds that result from the decomposition of these chemical agents—in the surrounding water and sediment to determine whether the chemicals pose a threat to human health or the environment. Seawater has likely eaten away at the metal containers, letting the compounds seep into the environment. According to some reports, the metal boxes holding the weapons may not have even been completely sealed to begin with. "In order to make these containers sink, they actually shot holes into them so that they would fill with seawater," Edwards says. "So between corrosion and the way these containers were handled at the surface there is certainly potential for leakage."

At this point, the team plans to avoid assessing the actual weapons and will only sample the surrounding seafloor and water—in large part a safety precaution because the weapons material could still be very dangerous. Exactly what happens to nerve agents and other chemical weapons once they sit in cold ocean water for decades is still not known. Seawater can dissolve and dilute the chemicals, but laboratory studies show that some chemical reactions break down these substances into different compounds, says Peter Brewer of the Monterey Bay Aquarium Research Institute in Moss Landing, Calif. "I suspect that the areas that are actually contaminated are probably quite small," he says.

Still, studies of a European dump site found that chemical mustard can form sticky nodules on bomb casings, trapping the intact chemical inside. "If you took those up to the surface and broke them, you could spill the mustard agent and cause serious burns," Edwards says. This scenario happened in 1976 when three scientists surveyed a dredge dump off the coast of Pearl Harbor and got burned when they accidentally recovered chemical weapons.

The team will publish all study results, Wilkens says. That's particularly important because the issue of chemical weapons in the oceans has been kept largely under wraps in many countries, Brewer says. "The topic has pretty much been a black hole." This secrecy has resulted in the injury of some 500 unsuspecting individuals, mostly fishermen who captured rotting chemical weapons in their nets. And among ocean scientists, "there is a huge lack of awareness of this issue," Brewer and Noriko Nakayama of the University of Tokyo wrote in a 2008 article in *Environmental Science & Technology*. Researchers routinely sample the water column in most of the known dumping areas, "often within a few meters of the seafloor" and "without regard for or knowledge of the disposed materials," the duo wrote. In the United States, for example, ocean scientists have conducted thousands of studies in a 10,400-square-kilometer territory off the coast of California that contains seven known dumping sites, Brewer says. But no one knows exactly where the weapons are.

Over the past few years, the U.S. Department of Defense has reviewed historical records to better understand the location of all chemical weapons that the U.S. military disposed of in U.S. coastal waters. But information is spotty: The records usually don't contain coordinates. In some cases, historical information only specifies "Atlantic Ocean" or "Pacific Ocean," according to a 2007 Congressional Research Service report.

The Hawaii Undersea Munitions and Material Assessment study could be a first step toward establishing procedures for how to search for and characterize deep-sea chemical weapons dump sites, says Vicki Gaynor, vice president of Environet, a company that works with the University of Hawaii. Because this site lies at moderate depth, only about 500 meters below the surface, it "gives the researchers a chance to test their technology and see how effective it is at really identifying what's out there," she says. At this point, however, no one really knows what to expect or even what the risks of surveying the dump site are, so the research team will include hazardous materials experts from the U.S. Army's Edgewood Chemical and Biological Center in Maryland. They will help design safety protocols, such as how to recover the submersibles and how to check them for any contamination before bringing the submersible on board or allowing anybody to get out. "We are on the cutting edge of doing this sort of thing," Edwards says, "so we are going to be learning as we go."

10

Iran May Seek Biological and Chemical Weapons

Jason Sigger

Jason Sigger is a defense policy analyst in the Washington, D.C. area. He writes about general military topics and specific chemical, biological, radiological, and nuclear (CBRN) defense issues, in addition to general day-to-day military issues.

While most analysts focus on Iran's nuclear program, some military strategists are also worried about the possibility of Iran acquiring or already stockpiling biological and chemical weapons. The country sustained much damage from Iraq's chemical weapons during the Iran-Iraq war of the 1980s, and it might feel compelled to safeguard itself by developing its own toxins and nerve agents. However, there's no conclusive evidence as to how far possible weapons programs have progressed, if they should indeed exist, making a coherent U.S. strategy extremely difficult.

The rest of the world may be focused on Iran's nuclear program. But U.S. intelligence agencies, think tanks, and non-governmental organizations just can't shake the suspicion that Iran may be trying to assemble other weapons of mass destruction, too: an arsenal of chemical and biological arms.

Anthony Cordesman, noted chemical-biological (CB) weapons and Middle East analyst for the Center for Strategic and International Studies, has released a few draft reports discussing the current capabilities and uncertainties of Iran's CB

Jason Sigger, "Chemical, Biological Arms: Iran's Other WMDs," Wired.com, October 29, 2008. Reproduced by permission of the author.

warfare programs. The papers offer a pretty good summary of what open-source analysis exists on "the other WMDs" that so many people tend to ignore, as the hysteria mounts about Iran's nuclear program.

Iran's government officials have both condemned CB weapons use, but also have noted that there could be incentives in having such a capability.

Iran's Complex Legacy

Iran is not an easy case to understand, to put it mildly. You may remember that minor conflict in the 1980s where Iraq attacked Iran and started throwing chemical weapons around. The chemical casualties incurred by Iran during that conflict was a major reason why Iran initiated its own chemical weapons program. Iran was an original state signatory to the Biological Weapons Convention in 1973 and signed onto the Chemical Weapons Convention in 1993. The country ratified the CWC in 1997 and declared its past program activities. This was followed by the destruction of Iran's former production sites in the presence of international arms control inspectors. Iran has also been very active in review conferences addressing biological weapons issues.

At the same time, U.S. observers still have a nagging feeling that Iran has been up to *something*. Here's the thing—Iran is a country with a modern industrial infrastructure and has been increasing its technological capabilities. The global economy, enhanced by global communications and transportation options, has benefited Iran just as much as any other growing nation. Russia and China, in particular, have been selling Iran equipment and material that could be used to develop CB weapons, but is legitimately used in commercial facilities and academic laboratories. Other nations have also been actively participating in the business of selling Iran materials and equipment. Given these facts, Iran has motive and opportunity to develop CB weapons—if its government wants that capability.

And while it *could be* that Iran's military desires and is pursuing a CB weapons capability, there is no public evidence of active development, testing, weaponization, stockpiling, deployment, or use of CB weapons. Without (at the least) evidence of testing and weaponization, it is very difficult to claim that Iran's military has a deployable capability to use CB weapons. Iran's government officials have both condemned CB weapons use, but also have noted that there could be incentives in having such a capability. US intelligence officials have, in open testimony, backed off of earlier claims in 2003 that Iran is *definitely developing and stockpiling* CB weapons to more conservative statements . . . this year that Iran has the *capability* to do so, and is suspected of engaging in CB weapons research and development. That's some significant backpedaling.

An Imperfect Argument

Cordesman doesn't offer much details in the form of suspected CB warfare agents or delivery systems, but he does generalize as to the possible. These case studies on agents and possible employment scenarios could apply to any nation with a modern industrial infrastructure, however. He doesn't offer any analysis as to the possibility of Iran supplying CB warfare agents to terrorists, other than to say, sure, it could happen. He ends his report on Iran's biological weapons program assessment with this statement, which is very similar to his conclusions about Tehran's chemical weapons programs:

> None of these problems and issues implies that Iran cannot benefit from deploying biological weapons or creating a level of ambiguity that forces any potential enemy to take these threats far more seriously than they are taken today. It

is also clear that Iran has the incentive to use biological weapons under some conditions and that such use might be effective.

Biological weapons also present special problems in terms of deterrence in peacetime and controlling escalation in a conflict. This does not mean that Iranian will act on the basis of ideology or ignore risk. Extreme as some Iranian statements are, Iran tends to be pragmatic in practice. Once again, however, crises create new conditions, perceptions, misunderstandings, and levels of risk taking.

Rational bargainers with perfect insight and all the necessary transparency in terms of full knowledge of the situation and risks are theoretical constructs. It is dangerous to assume that even the most prudent decision maker will not take exceptional risks, overreact, or drastically miscalculate in war.

That is to say, we really don't know what Iran has in the form of CB weapons or what they intend to do if it is given the opportunity to develop such weapons. And if that day comes when Iran's military does acknowledge that they have CB weapons, we really don't know what will happen, but they're not irrational leaders. Other than that, it's clear as day that we ought to at least consider the possibility.

11

North Korea Might Test Biological Weapons on Its Citizens

Gordon Chang

Gordon Chang is the author of Nuclear Showdown: North Korea Takes On the World, *which focuses on nuclear proliferation in general and the North Korean crisis in particular. His first book is* The Coming Collapse of China. *He is a columnist at Forbes.com.*

Although evidence against North Korea often relies on questionable sources, it has become apparent that the North Korean military uses its own people to test chemical and biological weapons. In the case of war, the North Korean government seems willing to use these weapons to defend its regime.

Is North Korea testing chemical and biological weapons on humans? The answer almost certainly is yes. Is it experimenting on children and the mentally handicapped? Probably so.

After decades of development, Pyongyang has stockpiled 2,500 to 5,000 tons of chemical weapons—mainly mustard gas, sarin, phosgene, and hydrogen cyanide—and is capable of rapid production in time of war. The arsenal, one of the world's largest, can be fired into South Korea either by artillery shell or with missiles.

When he was director of National Intelligence, John Negroponte cited the North's chemical weapons as among the

Gordon Chang, "Is North Korea Testing Biological Weapons on Children?" *Pajamas Media*, July 28, 2009. Reproduced by permission.

"greatest threats" to the United States. The North is believed to operate 12 facilities producing chemicals for war use.

North Korea has also weaponized anthrax, smallpox, pneumonic plague, cholera, and botulism and may have as many as 5,000 tons of biological agents. [North Korean leader] Kim Jong Il's militant state is thought to have at least 20 plants involved in developing and producing these weapons. The North's program started in the 1960s, and it has a high call on the nation's meager resources.

So far, there has been no documented use of North Korea's chemical or biological agents on foreigners, but that does not mean there have been no victims. Some, such as national security analyst John Loftus, think the high toll—perhaps 3,000 killed or injured—resulting from the train blast in Ryongchon, a town close to the China border, in April 2004 was the result of the release of chemical or biological agents being transported to Syria. That charge has never been proven.

More certain, however, are the accusations that North Korea has tested chemical and biological agents on its own people. "An officer ordered me to select 50 healthy female prisoners. One of the guards handed me a basket full of soaked cabbage, told me not to eat it but to give it to the fifty women," said Sun Ok Lee, a former prisoner, in the middle of this decade. "All who ate the cabbage leaves started violently vomiting blood and screaming with pain. It was hell. In less than 20 minutes they were quite dead."

A General Lack of Evidence

None of the allegations, including Lee's, can be substantiated. All of them come from refugees and defectors, who have a general motive to make their stories appear of great value to South Korean and Western intelligence agencies. As a result of the incentive to fabricate, some of what we hear from those fleeing Kim's state is almost certainly untrue.

For example, Pyongyang—and some of its harshest critics—allege that the BBC 2004 program *Access to Evil*, which reported that chemical weapons were used on political prisoners, relied on faked North Korean documents. The documents—orders to transfer prisoners for the purpose of experimentation—could be forgeries because they carry seals that do not look genuine.

North Korea is not only testing chemical and biological weapons, it is also rehearsing their use.

Yet even if some defector stories are untrue, fleeing North Koreans, over time, have told essentially the same story, thereby unintentionally corroborating each other. For instance, Kwon Hyok, formerly the chief of security at the now-infamous Camp 22, states that small groups of people were led into a chamber with glass windows and suffocated with gas while technicians observed the gruesome process. Compare this to the testimony of Im Chun-yong, a former North Korean commando. He says one of his soldiers told him of a facility on an island off the country's west coast where people were put into a glass chamber. "Poisonous gas was injected in," Im says, relating the story secondhand. "He watched doctors time how long it took for them to die."

A Widespread Practice

Kim Sang-hun says that when he was a UN official he had interviewed hundreds of fleeing citizens, and most of them talked about the horrifying testing. "Human experimentation is a widespread practice," he notes.

Im, once a captain in Brigade No. 19, a special forces unit, confirms the experimentation is commonplace and also alleges that the government uses mentally and physically handicapped children, relating the story of his commander, who was essentially forced to give up his 12-year-old mentally ill daughter in the early 1990s. There may be as many as five locations where such testing takes place, says Kim, the former UN official.

North Korea is not only testing chemical and biological weapons, it is also rehearsing their use. Im said he was given training on firing a "bazooka-style" weapon delivering WMD.

Would North Korea actually use its chemical and biological weapons? Im, for one, is convinced Kim Jong Il would not hesitate to do so. The country, after all, is run by ruthless men and women who have committed horrific acts in the past. Killing their own citizens, especially the handicapped, is consistent with all we know about the criminals responsible for the most abhorrent regime on earth today.

Organizations to Contact

The editors have compiled the following list of organizations concerned with the issues debated in this book. The descriptions are derived from materials provided by the organizations. All have publications or information available for interested readers. The list was compiled on the date of publication of the present volume; the information provided here may change. Readers need to remember that many organizations take several weeks or longer to respond to inquiries.

**British American Security Information Council
(BASIC UK)**
The Grayston Centre, 2nd Floor, London   N1 6HT
    United Kingdom
+44 (0) 20 7324 4680
Web site: www.basicint.org

BASIC is a progressive and independent analysis and advocacy organization that researches and provides a critical examination of global security issues, including nuclear policies, military strategies, armaments, and disarmament. BASIC assists in the development of global security policies, policy-making, and the assessment of policy priorities, and it promotes public awareness and understanding of these policies and of policy-making in Europe and the United States. Articles on biological warfare and bio-defense are available on its Web site.

The Brookings Institution
1775 Massachusetts Ave. NW, Washington, DC   20036
(202) 797-6000 • fax: (202) 797-6004
E-mail: brookinfo@brook.edu
Web site: www.brookings.edu

The Brookings Institution is a think tank conducting research and education in foreign policy, economics, government, and the social sciences. Publications include periodic *Policy Briefs* and books including *Terrorism and U.S. Foreign Policy.*

Center for Defense Information (CDI)
1779 Massachusetts Ave. NW, Washington, DC   20036
(202) 332-0600 • fax: (202) 462-4559
E-mail: info@cdi.org
Web site: www.cdi.org

CDI is a nonpartisan, nonprofit organization that researches all aspects of global security. It seeks to educate the public and policy makers about weapons systems, security policy, and defense budgeting. It publishes the monthly *Defense Monitor*.

Center for Strategic and International Studies (CSIS)
1800 K Street NW, Washington, DC   20006
(202) 887-0200 • fax: (202) 775-3199
Web site: www.csis.org

The center works to provide world leaders with strategic insights and policy options on current and emerging global issues. It publishes the *Washington Quarterly*, a journal on political, economic, and security issues, and other publications that can be downloaded from its Web site.

Central Intelligence Agency (CIA)
Office of Public Affairs, Washington, DC   20505
(703) 482-0623 • fax: (703) 482-1739
Web site: www.cia.gov

The Central Intelligence Agency was created in 1947 with the signing of the National Security Act by President Harry S. Truman. The CIA seeks to collect and evaluate intelligence related to the national security and provide appropriate dissemination of such intelligence. Publications such as the *Factbook on Intelligence* are available on its Web site.

Federation of American Scientists (FAS)
1725 DeSales Street NW, 6th Floor, Washington, DC   20036
(202) 546-3300 • fax: (202) 675-1010
E-mail: fas@fas.org
Web site: www.fas.org

The Federation of American Scientists' Biological and Chemical Weapons Control Project covers all aspects of chemical and biological weapons and their control, but it concentrates on researching and advocating policies that balance science and security without harming national security or scientific progress. FAS seeks to prevent the misuse of its members' research and to promote public understanding of the real threats from biological and chemical weapons. FAS publishes information on biological and chemical weapons online, as well as fact sheets on anthrax, cyanide, and other toxins.

The Heritage Foundation
214 Massachusetts Ave. NE, Washington, DC   20002-4999
(202) 546-4400 • fax: (202) 546-8328
E-mail: info@heritage.org
Web site: www.heritage.org

Founded in 1973, the Heritage Foundation is a research and educational institute. Its mission is to formulate and promote conservative public policies based on the principles of free enterprise, limited government, individual freedom, and a strong national defense. It publishes many books on foreign policy, such as *Winning the Long War*.

National Security Agency (NSA)
9800 Savage Road, Fort Meade, MD   20755-6248
(301) 688-6524
Web site: www.nsa.gov

The NSA coordinates, directs, and performs activities, such as designing cipher systems, that protect American information systems and produce foreign intelligence information. Speeches, briefings, and reports are available online.

United Nations Foundation
1800 Massachusetts Ave. NW, Suite 400
Washington, DC   20036
(202) 887-9040

E-mail unwire@unfoundation.org
Web site: www.unfoundation.org

The foundation's daily news summary covers the United Nations, global affairs, and key international issues. UN Wire provides a concise, daily summary of key news stories from around the world. UN Wire also features direct, immediate links to full-text, audio, video, and additional sources of information on the Internet.

World Health Organization (WHO) Epidemic and Pandemic Alert and Response
Avenue Appia 20, Geneva 27 1211
  Switzerland
+41 (0) 22 791 2111
Web site: www.who.int/csr/en

The World Health Organization is the United Nations specialized agency for health. WHO's global alert and response activities and the Outbreak Alert and Response Network are aimed at the detection, verification, and containment of epidemics. In the event of the intentional release of a biological agent, these activities could be vital to international containment efforts. Access to publications such as the *World Health Report* can be had via the organization's Web site.

Bibliography

Books

Francis Anthony Boyle · *Biowarfare and Terrorism*. Atlanta, GA: Clarity Press, 2005.

Frederic Joseph Brown · *Chemical Warfare: A Study in Restraints*. New Brunswick, NJ: Transaction Publishers, 2006.

Anthony Cordesman · *The Challenge of Biological Terrorism: When to "Cry Wolf," What to Cry, and How to Cry It*. Washington, DC: CSIS, 2005.

Malcolm Dando · *Bioterror and Biowarfare: A Beginner's Guide*. Oxford, England: Oneworld Publications, 2006.

Richard Danzig · *After an Attack: Preparing Citizens for Bioterrorism*. Washington, DC: Center for a New American Security, 2007.

Thanos Dokos · *Countering the Proliferation of Weapons of Mass Destruction: NATO and EU Options in the Mediterranean and the Middle East*. New York: Routledge, 2008.

David Fidler · *Biosecurity in the Global Age: Biological Weapons, Public Health and the Rule of Law*. Stanford, CA: Stanford Law and Politics, 2008.

Stephen Flanagan and James Schear, eds.   *Strategic Challenges: America's Global Security Agenda.* Washington, DC: National Defense University Press, 2008.

I.W. Fong and Kenneth Alibek   *Bioterrorism and Infectious Agents: A New Dilemma for the 21st Century.* New York, Springer, 2005.

Benjamin Garrett and John Hart   *Historical Dictionary of Nuclear, Biological, and Chemical Warfare.* Lanham, MD: Scarecrow Press, 2007.

Karl Taro Greenfeld   *China Syndrome: The True Story of the 21st Century's First Great Epidemic.* New York: HarperCollins, 2006.

Jeanne Guillemin   *Biological Weapons: From the Invention of State-Sponsored Programs to Contemporary Bioterrorism.* New York: Columbia University Press, 2005.

Alexander Kelle et al.   *Controlling Biochemical Weapons: Adapting Multilateral Arms Control for the 21st Century.* New York: Palgrave, 2006.

Alexander Kouzminov   *Biological Espionage: Special Operations of the Soviet and Russian Foreign Intelligence Services in the West.* Mechanicsburg, PA: Stackpole Books, 2005.

Milton Leitenberg   *Assessing the Biological Weapons and Bioterrorism Threat.* Carlisle Barracks, PA: Strategic Studies Institute, 2005.

Jez Littlewood   *The Biological Weapons Convention: A Failed Revolution.* Burlington, VT: Ashgate, 2005.

Christopher Mari, ed.   *Global Epidemics.* New York: H.W. Wilson Company, 2007.

National Research Council   *Combined Exposures to Hydrogen Cyanide and Carbon Monoxide in Army Operations: Initial Report.* Washington, DC: National Academies Press, 2008.

National Research Council   *Globalization, Biosecurity, and the Future of the Life Sciences.* Washington, DC: National Academies Press, 2006.

National Research Council   *Sensor Systems for Biological Agent Attacks: Protecting Buildings and Military Bases.* Washington, DC: National Academy Press, 2005.

Thomas Preston   *From Lambs to Lions: Future Security Relationships in a World of Biological and Nuclear Weapons.* Lanham, MD: Rowman & Littlefield, 2007.

Sergey Rumyantsev   *Biological Weapon: A Terrible Reality? Profound Delusion? Skillful Swindling?* New York: Vantage Press, 2006.

James Russell and James Wirtz   *Globalization and WMD Proliferation: Terrorism, Transnational Networks, and International Security.* New York: Routledge, 2008.

Philipp Sarasin   *Anthrax: Bioterror as Fact and Fantasy.* Cambridge, MA: Harvard University Press, 2006.

Fred Stone   *The "Worried Well" Response to CBRN Events: Analysis and Solutions.* Maxwell Air Force Base, AL: USAF Counterproliferation Center, Air University, 2007.

Ramesh Thakur and Ere Haru, eds.   *The Chemical Weapons Convention: Implementation, Challenges and Opportunities.* New York: UN University Press, 2006.

George Whitbred   *Offensive Use of Chemical Technologies by US Special Operations Forces in the Global War on Terrorism: The Nonlethal Option.* Maxwell Air Force Base, AL: Air War College, Air University, 2006.

Geoffrey Zubay, ed.   *Agents of Bioterrorism: Pathogens & Their Weaponization.* New York: Columbia University Press, 2005.

Periodicals

Kyle Ballard   "Convention in Peril? Riot Control Agents and the Chemical Weapons Ban," *Arms Control Today*, September 2007.

Sergey Batsanov   "Approaching the 10th Anniversary of the Chemical Weapons Convention: A Plan for Future Progress," *Nonproliferation Review*, July 2006.

Rita Boland — "Biological Sensor Detects Hazards," *Signal*, April 2006.

John Borrie — "The Limits of Modest Progress: The Rise, Fall, and Return of Efforts to Strengthen the Biological Weapons Convention," *Arms Control Today*, October 2006.

Bureau of Industry and Security — U.S. Department of Commerce, "Chemical Weapons Convention: Sampling and Analysis," *Chemical Weapons Convention Bulletin*, 2006.

Christopher Chyba — "Biotechnology and the Challenge to Arms Control," *Arms Control Today*, October 2006.

Rex Coppom — "Defending Against Bioterrorism," *Military Engineer*, January–February 2006.

Matthew Daily — "Senators Decry Plan to Transport Chemical Weapons," Associated Press, July 9, 2008.

Chris Doane and Joe DiRenzo — "NBC (Nuclear, Biological, and Chemical) Weapons of Mass Destruction: Detection, Warning, Protection and Countermeasures," *Naval Forces*, 2007.

Brian Ferguson — "Finding the Nerve," *Airman*, Spring 2007.

Mark Hewish — "SAIC Leads Team for US Army CBRN Protection System," *Jane's International Defense Review*, July 2004.

Spencer Hsu   "U.S. Bioterrorism Efforts Criticized,"
                     Washington Post, October 22, 2009.

Donna Hudson   "Counter-Biological Warfare
                     Initiatives," *TIG Brief*, Summer 2006.

Kate Ivanova and   "CBRN Attack Perpetrators: An
Todd Sandler   Empirical Study," *Foreign Policy
                     Analysis*, October 2007.

Hunter Keeter   "CBRN Defence—Still Required After
                     the Demise of the East-West
                     Confrontation?" *Naval Forces*, 2005.

Kelly Kennedy   "Studies Link Gulf War Illnesses to
                     Sarin Gas," *Navy Times*, June 25,
                     2007.

Roger Lane   "NATO Transformation: The
                     Development of a CBRN
                     (Chemical-Biological-Radiological-Nuclear)
                     Defence Capability," *RUSI Journal*,
                     August 2004.

Tom McCreery   "Defence Against Biological,
and Wayne   Chemical and Radiological Attacks:
Bryden   The Technological Way Forward,"
                     Military Technology, 2006.

Mark McDonald   "C-CBRNE (Counter-Chemical,
                     Biological, Radiological, Nuclear and
                     High-Yield Explosive) ETE:
                     Education, Training and Exercise,"
                     TIG Brief, Fall 2006.

Albert Mauroni   "The Future of Chemical, Biological,
                     Radiological, and Nuclear Defense,"
                     Joint Force Quarterly, January 2007.

Larry Neumeister and Devlin Barrett — "Uncle Follows Nephew to NYC for Terror Trial," Associated Press, November 24, 2009.

New York Times — "Chemical Weapons Watchdog Pursues Holdout Nations," *New York Times*, December 3, 2009.

Wendy Orent — "Our Own Worst Bioenemy," *Los Angeles Times*, August 13, 2008.

Tim Otter — "Supply and Demand: Keeping End-Users in Mind Fosters Effective CBRN (Chemical, Biological, Radiological, Nuclear) Defence," *Jane's International Defense Review*, August 2007.

Barry Rosenberg — "See No Evil: Countering WMD Proliferation Is a Job the Pentagon Doesn't Want," *Armed Forces Journal*, May 2007.

Argie Sarantinos-Perrin — "Eliminating Chemical Weapons," *Soldiers*, March 2007.

Tony Skinner — "Briefing: NATO CBRN (Chemical, Biological, Radiological or Nuclear) Capabilities," *Jane's Defence Weekly*, March 5, 2008.

Gareth Smith — "Why Iran's Revolutionary Guards Mercilessly Crack Down," *Christian Science Monitor*, August 6, 2009.

James Tegnelia — "A New Era in Combating WMD," *Joint Force Quarterly*, March 2007.

Breanne Wagner   "Buried Poison: Abandoned
                  Chemical Weapons Pose Continual
                  Threat," *National Defense*, August
                  2007.

Clyde Ward   "Fitz Harber Said of His Chemical
                  Agents, Especially Mustard Gas, 'It Is
                  a Higher Form of Killing,'" *Military
                  History*, May 2006.

Index

Loftus, John, 78
Louisiana, 39

M

Maine, 39
Maryland, 39, 66, 72
Matsumoto, Chizuo, 18
Maurer, Stephen, 55–60
Mauroni, Al, 33–36
Montana, 39
Monterey Bay Aquarium Research Institute, 71
Monterey Institute of International Studies, 63
Mossad organization (Israel), 16
Musgrave, David, 62
Mustard gas, 8, 62, 69, 71, 77

N

Nakayama, Noriko, 71
National Academy of Sciences, 66
National Defense, 9
Nazif, Dana, 8
Nebraska, 39
Negroponte, John, 77
New Hampshire, 39
Nobel Prize, 16
Nonstockpile materiel, 9
North Carolina, 39
North Korea, 77–80
Nuclear weapons, 34–35
Nunn, Sam, 29

O

Obama, Barack, 27, 32, 33–34, 62, 67
Ocean as weapon dumping site, 9, 68–72

Oklahoma, 29
Oklahoma City bombing, 22
OPCW (Organization for the Prohibition of Chemical Weapons), 10
Oppenheimer, Andy, 10–14
Oregon, 18–19, 66
O'Toole, Tara, 26–30, 31
Ouagrham-Gormley, Sonia Ben, 40–54

P

Palestine, 16, 35
Pentagon, 20, 66
Personal protective equipment (PPE), 13
Pharmaceutical stockpiles, 17, 24
Phosgene, 77
Plague
    anti-plague system, 40–54
    plague bacteria, 20, 24, 38, 78
Poisoned arrows/spears, 7
Pueblo Chemical Depot, 67

Q

Quadrennial Defense Review, 33

R

Rajneesh, Bhagwan Shree, 19
Reagan, Ronald, 65
Recession, 37–39
Red Army Faction (Germany), 16
Red Brigades (Italy), 16
Ricin, 20
Rightist groups, 15, 17, 19–20, 22
Russia, 43, 53, 74. *See also* Soviet Union
Rutgers University, 32